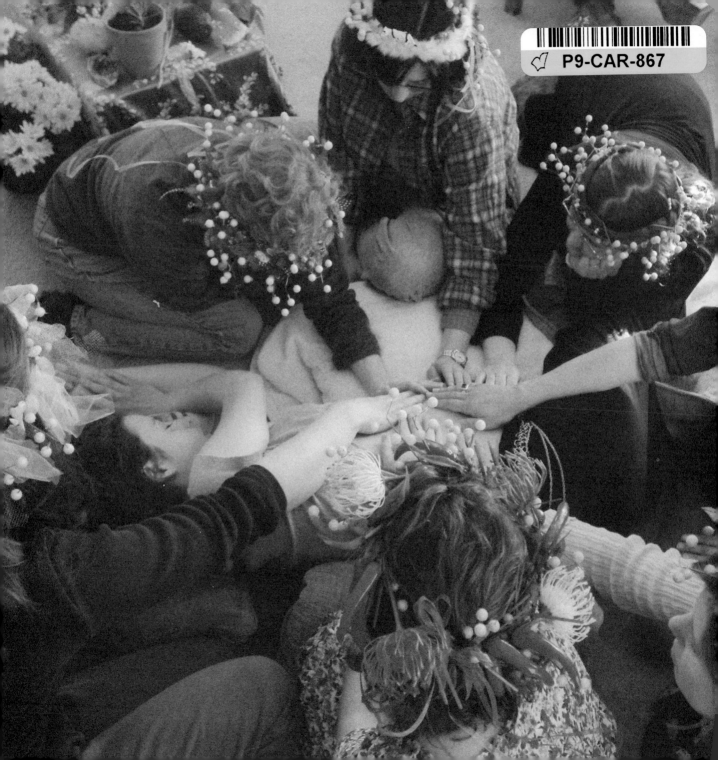

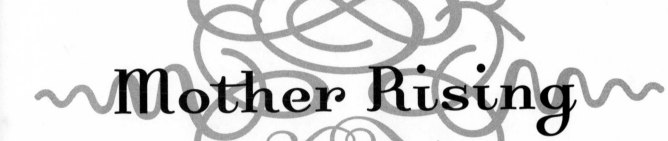

Mother Rising

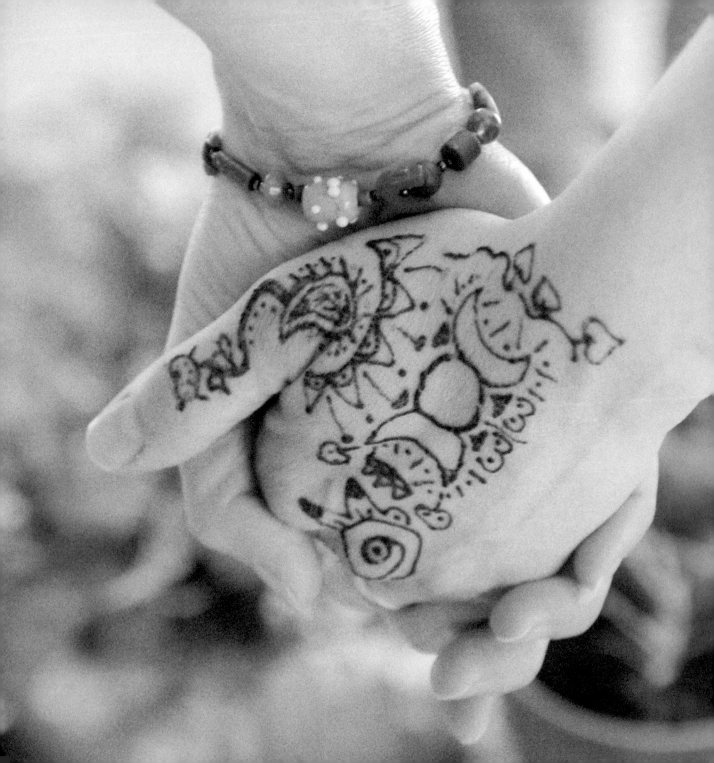

Mother Rising

The Blessingway Journey
into Motherhood

Yana Cortlund ❀ Barb Lucke ❀ Donna Miller Watelet

CELESTIAL ARTS
Berkeley | Toronto

First published by Seeing Stone Press

Library of Congress Cataloging-in-Publication Data
Cortlund, Yana.
 Mother rising : the blessingway journey into motherhood /
Yana Cortlund, Barb Lucke, and Donna Miller Watelet.
  p. cm.
  Includes bibliographical references and index.
 ISBN-13: 978-1-58761-267-1 (pbk.)
 ISBN-10: 1-58761-267-4 (pbk.)
 1. Motherhood—Miscellanea. 2. Birth customs.
 3. Self-help groups. I. Lucke, Barb.
 II. Watelet, Donna Miller. III. Title.

 HQ759.C7454 2006
 392.1'2—dc22   2006007790

Printed in the United States of America
First printing, 2006
1 2 3 4 5 6 7 8 9 10—10 09 08 07 06

Distributed in Australia by Simon and Schuster Australia, in Canada by Ten Speed Press Canada, in New Zealand by Southern Publishers Group, in South Africa by Real Books, and in the United Kingdom and Europe by Airlift Book Company.

Cover design by Dorothy Marschall based on an original design by Yana Cortlund and Tanya Olsen
Text design by Dorothy Marschall
Circle symbol illustrations by Ann Miya

The authors of gratefully acknowledge permission to reprint the following: Adaptation of "Prayer for Clarity," by Shea Darian, from *Seven Times the Sun* © 2001, reprinted by permission of Gilead Press. Adaptation of material excerpted from *Celebrating Motherhood: A Comforting Companion for Every Expecting Mother* by Andrea Alban Gosline, Lisa Burnett Bossi, Ame Mahler Beanland with permission of Conari Press, an imprint of Red Wheel/Weiser, Boston, MA, and York Beach, ME.

Celestial Arts
Box 7123
Berkeley, California 94707
www.tenspeed.com

DEDICATION

For our children: Sean, Carly, Evan, Claire, and Lyra—
because without you, we wouldn't be here.

ON THE DAY OF THE BLESSINGWAY, we arrive like flowing water: first a trickle, then a stream. Soon, our current builds to that of a great river, and by the time the last one of us has come, gathered together, we create a vast and powerful sea. As we drop our bags and smooth our flowing skirts, a bell chimes. Silence descends as we quiet our bodies and our minds.

We line up from eldest to youngest, and one by one we are smudged by a beautifully adorned woman who holds burning herbs and a feathered fan in her hand. We dip our fingers into rose-scented water, release our lingering cares, then walk into the sacred space that has been set for the blessingway. Circle formed, we stand, quietly swaying to soft music. Once the youngest of the women has joined us, we are led in prayer to cast our circle, then invited to be seated.

Elemental energies are evoked all around; the Goddess is called to the center. Together as one, we begin to sing: our music connecting us to the center of ourselves, to each other, to Spirit. We are guided to empty our expectations and fears into the flames that create space for the work to come.

As we let go, we fall softly into a state of sweet reverie. We gently lead the mother-to-be to a grand seat, a place of power and of honor. Here she is bathed, she is caressed, and with loving hands, she is made ready for her journey…

CONTENTS

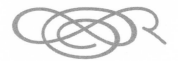

FOREWORD

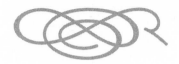

IT IS OFTEN SAID that what Western culture needs more now than ever are rituals to mark important transitions in our status. In fact, it is not that we need rituals more now; conscious, socialized human beings have always needed rituals! For many reasons, celebrations of birth as a sacred rite of passage in the West have been absent for too long.

Somewhere inside every woman is a deep knowing, even if it is barely conscious, that giving birth is a multi-layered, mysterious rite of passage. Many women realize it only after they give birth, in private moments when they reflect on what happened to them and within them. It is then they secretly wish that they had been prepared differently—that in some way they had honored the event that would completely change their mind, body, and soul. This wish often turns to grief, and then is gradually forgotten as caring for the baby consumes their life.

Whether they realize it or not, everyone—parents, babies, and birth professionals—is feeling the wounding impact of the ritual of childbirth preparation having been reduced to medical orientation. In recent years there have been rebellious ripples of remembering that birth is a sacred rite of passage; an increasing number of courageous and creative women have modified or abandoned baby showers altogether to experiment with blessingways that honor the mother.

The parched, ritual-thirsty soul of society is calling for a change. In the absence of tradition and elders, we desperately need new direction. I applaud the authors of *Mother Rising* for answering that call. I cannot praise the authors enough for their voice and vision. *Mother Rising* gives our generation the sweet, nourishing nectar to inspire the creation of rich, soulful, memorable blessingways that bless not only the mother, but every participant and, ultimately, everyone in society.

A woman's experience in birth and the outcome of her birth is influenced by a vast web of influences. We see only a fraction of the threads that make up the fabric of a birth. It is influenced not only by what the mother eats, but what her mind and soul is fed from the time she is playing with dolls until the day she is in labor. It is mysterious and complex.

We are led to believe birth outcome is largely determined by "prenatal care" or safe medical management; that belief has made us as a community of women incredibly passive and disconnected. While it is true we cannot absolutely control the outcome of a birth, we must not believe that we are not without power or influence.

Even if you have never led a sacred ceremony, by following the clear guidance in *Mother Rising*, you will have the confidence to do it. Make the space, gather the people, bring your intention; the ceremony itself has power and makes the magic happen.

It is within every one of us to make a difference. We can't wait until we know how, or hope someone else will do it. More powerful than your experience, it is your loving, positive intention that will move the mother, open her, ground her, and enrich her in ways you cannot imagine.

This is a groundbreaking book. *Mother Rising* is expertly and warmly written and well-organized. Each page draws you in, and slowly draws out of you indigenous, soulful wisdom and confidence you never knew you had. When blessingway rituals become a Western tradition, birth outcomes will change.

—Pam England, CNM, MA,
coauthor of *Birthing from Within*

PREFACE

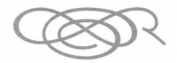

THE IDEAS PRESENTED in *Mother Rising* began to take form over fifteen years ago when Barb, then a new mother, began attending La Leche League meetings. (La Leche League [LLL] is an international organization whose mission is to help mothers breastfeed through mother-to-mother support, encouragement, information, and education.) During those monthly LLL gatherings, she found the support, the connection, and the understanding she so desperately needed as a new mother in transition.

In the company of a women's circle that grew out of her La Leche League affiliation, Barb was introduced to the concept of blessingways, and she soon began planning them herself. As her knowledge and experience as a ritual leader grew, more and more women began approaching her for ceremonies and information, and her folder of notes grew fat with possibility.

As her own children grew and began school, Barb recognized the need to support herself through this new transitional stage of motherhood, and she formed another women's circle. There, she continued her work with Yana and Donna, and together they shared and entrusted the details of their lives, emotions, questions, and answers with one another over the next five years.

Still, the book you hold in your hands might never have come about if not for a single event. Barb was preparing to go into a month-long meditative retreat just when two members of the LLL group she led at the time expressed interest in having blessingways. Yana, who had attended two blessingways (one of them her own), volunteered to plan the events in Barb's absence, and Barb handed over her folder of notes.

Faced with someone else's pile of random scribbles, paper scraps, partial thoughts, and bits and pieces of this and that, Yana began sifting through to unearth the essence of the ceremony. In studying this collection of blessingway invitations and various ritual outlines, she uncovered visionary ideas, inspiring quotes, and beautiful musings.

By the time Barb returned from retreat, Yana was overflowing with enthusiasm and ideas of her own. The two decided to put down on paper a simple guide to creating blessingways. Because of their individual skill sets, they divided up project tasks and went off to work on their own. But before long, they became overwhelmed, frustrated, and lonely. The project began to feel heavy. What was wrong?

They realized they had lost sight of the most essential element of their project: the power of women coming together. It had been clear to them from the start that this book was not one that could be written alone by a single author, nor should it be, given its core message. So they reached out to involve other women.

Yana and Barb's need for research help and their questions about spirituality led them to approach Donna, an interfaith minister trained to serve people of all faiths and spiritual paths. With her many years of experience creating and leading rituals, Donna quickly became a valuable addition to their team. She soon put her knowledge and skills to work making *Mother Rising* accessible to any woman who chooses the blessingway journey, honoring these women's own beliefs, and finding the connections and language to bridge them together.

❀ . ❀ . ❀

We, the core members of what is now a collective, began *Mother Rising* as individuals. But we were brought together by more than just circumstance. We came together by the hands of divine inspiration, and—above all—a belief that women's wisdom is worth preserving, celebrating, and sharing.

Over the course of four and a half years, we have come to understand that this work is much larger than we are ourselves, and we know that it will continue on even if some of us should drop away from it. *Mother Rising* is the progeny of our union, stronger and more complete than any one of us could have created on her own.

Our book completed, would we now call ourselves experts or authorities on women's blessingway rituals?

We are perhaps more accurately archivists and historians. We are collectors and weavers of women's work. We are mothers; we are teachers; we are storytellers.

We are American women looking for our own culturally alive, modern expression of life's most profound experiences, beginning with how we prepare to give birth to our babies. We are just like you in many ways. So we've written down what we know so far, and—as it was passed on to us—we now pass it on to you.

ACKNOWLEDGMENTS

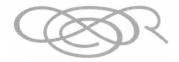

IT HAS BEEN OUR MANTRA all along to put our families first. Thus we have learned to weave our work around their needs. During this book project, we often found ourselves typing with one hand while nursing infants; reading books on ritual while waiting to pick up carloads of kids; and frantically jotting down important concepts on the back of grocery lists in the middle of the canned food aisle.

Throughout our journey, one of the most essential lessons we learned was that our daily lives were, in fact, integral to the work we were doing. Events that, at first glance, appeared to be delays, detours, and interruptions consistently revealed themselves to be project-enriching gifts—for when we returned to the work at hand, we did so with new perspectives, greater insights, and far more open hearts.

We do, however, recognize that our involvement in this work has added stress to our home lives, and we honor and thank our families for giving us not only the leeway, but also the encouragement necessary to pursue and finish this book.

We are all especially grateful for the assistance of Yana's dad, Alex Cortlund, for his belief in us and in our project. His financial investment in this book took the form of hiring a nanny to care for Yana's children, freeing up a few precious hours a day for her. Without his support, the time needed to write this book would never have been created. Thank you so much, Alex!

As our project progressed and gained momentum, we found that providence (in the form of many friends and family members) stepped in at all the right moments. Judy Wolf offered her time and editing skills; Kathleen Cortlund, Helen Lutz, Samantha McCall, and Laurie Riedman read the initial manuscript and provided valuable feedback; Jason Cortlund, Dave Feasey, Sue Feasey, Lynn Barnett, Lynn Malooly, and Vanessa Brown proofread the final draft of the book and verified the index; and Tanya Olsen created the cover and text design for the original version of *Mother Rising*, published by Seeing Stone Press in 2004.

Many women embraced *Mother Rising* immediately upon its initial publication, and we would especially like to thank both Pam England and Suzanne Arms for their respective support and encouragement.

Finally, we are very aware that our union as a collective has been divinely inspired, therefore we would be negligent if we did not thank and honor all the expressions of the Divine who aligned their efforts to first bring us together, and have since guided us on our journey to discovering and passing on this knowledge.

BARB'S ACKNOWLEDGMENTS

To La Leche League and the seven women I met there who formed a play group twelve years ago: It was through you that I was introduced to the concept of a blessingway, and we went on to discover the magic of ritual together. We have done many rituals together, helped birth each other's babies, and, most important, continued to gather together monthly to share good food and the joys and sorrows in our lives. Thanks Mary Joan, Lynn B., Lynn M., Nora, Susan, Donna G., and Anne for being my cheerleaders, inspiration, and, at times, my lifeline.

To Yana, Donna, and Tanya: thanks for answering the call to do this work. I am so aware that our union with each other has been divinely inspired—each one of us carrying unique gifts and talents that have been not only integral to, but down right magical in the creation of this book and the ritual work that we do. Not one of us could have accomplished this alone. Together we make up the four points on the compass, and together we will always find our way through life's sometimes rough seas.

To my husband, Mike: thanks for thinking that what we were up to was way cool. I think this email that you wrote really sums up how you feel about the work we are doing:

> It is easy to be light, truthful, and supportive of you because . . . I see your beauty, humility, and sweet-easy-coolness. When I saw you reading *Ya Ya [Sisterhood]*, sprawled in the back of Cool Mama Number Two's tie-dye mobile, I was struck by you and the scene—child-like goddesses just play'n with all the creative power of the cosmos—right there at my gas station. I would have loved to climb in and soak up the red pepper and sweet potato energy, yumm. Where're we going, girlfriends?

I love that this is how you see us, and know you wish you could be a part of our inner women's world! Your enthusiastic support of me and this project carries me when I myself am doubting or fearful. You have continually been my guide into the realm of joy, fun, and pleasure. Thank you for giving me the support to explore and pursue what I am passionate about.

To my son, Sean: I owe you the biggest heap of gratitude, for without having gone through the experience of bringing you into this world and learning the joyous lessons of surrender, love, and service through being your mommy, I am certain that I would never have crossed the threshold that landed me amidst the circles of amazing women who have led me to do this work. Honestly, I owe it all to you.

To my daughter, Carly: I am indebted to you for teaching me that no matter what hardships you face, being happy is always an option. I know that you have a lifetime worth of lessons to teach me. You are my shining light . . . and yes, you can work with us when you grow up.

YANA'S ACKNOWLEDGMENTS

To my parents, Alex and Kathleen Cortlund: Dad, thank you for not only being an extraordinary father, but for being my good friend as well. I feel so blessed to have your love, guidance, trust, and support. Your wholehearted belief in me gives me the courage to keep pursuing my dreams, especially during uncertain times. Thanks especially for always making sure that I have everything I need to live a happy life, as well as your encouragement and wise counsel to write anything, as long

as it's the truth. Kathleen, thank you for being the best mom a gal like me could ever have. The depth of your awareness, your loving care, and the genuine interest you take in my life makes me feel very supported in everything that I do. You are an incredibly wise woman whom I hope to work with on future projects. Thanks for listening, and even more, for always asking me the question, *"So how are you doing?"*

To my husband, Dave: thank you for your love and support, and for encouraging me way back when to find my own personal path to Spirit. I thank you as well for our two beautiful (though unceasingly energetic) daughters, our morning talks on the couch, making the coffee, answering zillions of hardware and software questions, and very importantly—though times have been quite tough—for resisting the temptation to tell me that I need to go out and get a paying job.

To my daughters, Lyra and Claire: thanks for helping me open my heart to Spirit and to this work. I love that at four and six years old, you both nurse your baby dolls, know what a blessingway is, and want to grow up just so you can ride a broomstick. And when five o'clock comes—and I'm still typing away—thank you for coming into my office, tugging on my arm, and saying, *"Mom, it's time to be with us!"*

To my good friend, Cliff Launt: I am so grateful for your spiritual guidance, support, and encouragement. My life just wouldn't be the same without our weekly Ghost Dances, meditations, and healings. So a great big thanks for showing up on my doorstep that night long ago with your stack of papers, as well as for generously providing me with the plethora of spiritual accoutrements necessary to walking this path. I am also thankful for the free, unlimited access to your CD collection!

My deepest gratitude and many, many thanks to Barb, Donna, and Tanya, for constantly reminding me of the value of my gifts and of the powerful force of the collective feminine spirit. Thanks for being open to unconventional ways and means, for laughing at my peculiar sense of humor, and for showing me that there is indeed magic in the world. Never before have I had friendships of such depth. I look forward to the years ahead of us, for there is much work for us yet to do.

DONNA'S ACKNOWLEDGMENTS

Many thanks to my preachers and teachers, who opened my mind and heart to deeper ways of connecting with others and celebrating life: Rev. Hans Klee, Diane McNally, John Mincher, Bill Stark, Kitty Macy, Kay Lynn Sullivan, Rabbi Joseph Gelberman, and S. S. Hari Simran Kaur Khalsa. Your willingness to show me the way to the present through the wisdom of the past is my greatest gift.

A very love-filled thank you to my son, Evan, who is such a light and a beacon of joy and wisdom in my life. You are my Buddha boy, teaching me lessons of love, patience, and giving. You graciously share me with the other people I work with. I love you very much, Evan. And I am so grateful to your father. Luc, your never-flagging support of this book made it possible for me to immerse myself in this wonderful work and allow it to flow and grow. Thank you so much.

My thanks to my parents and my family for their depth and light: my mother, Lois Miller, who lives life with God out in the open and who loved me through all it took for me to find my wings; my father, Bill Miller, whose booming humor makes me laugh and whose reverence for the beauty of this earth taught me to love and protect nature, and to be inspired by it; my older brother, Keith, my childhood pal, whose brilliance and friendship make my world shine so brightly; my high school girlfriend, Jane, my first real sister, who married my brother and is a role model mom for me, and whose teaching is a sacred gift; my younger brother, Dale, my six-foot-tall little buddy, an old soul with an incredible mind and heart, who inspired me from his earliest days with his deep wisdom that was always beyond his years. I love you all!

Special thanks to the many wise women in my family, all of whom enjoyed fulfilling work outside their homes, and also loved and cared for their families with open-hearted generosity: my dynamic cousin, Ellen Sue Dickinson; my courageous and caring aunts, Gloria Rowson and Dorothy Roth; and my inspiringly strong grand-mothers, Ruth Treichler and Dorothy Tread-well. Each of them showed me the deep beauty and grace of a woman who truly knows her power and uses it for love and goodness.

And finally, I'd like to give my most heart-felt thanks for the presence of three of the most remarkable women in my life. Barb, Yana, and Tanya, who are women of great vision, wisdom, courage, and brilliance, who inspire me with all that they are, to be everything that I can be. I am in awe of the grand design that gave us the opportunity to work together. And I am blessed beyond measure that these women chose to rise to this occasion with me. Thank you all for everything! The best is yet to come.

CHAPTER 1

Creating
New
Traditions

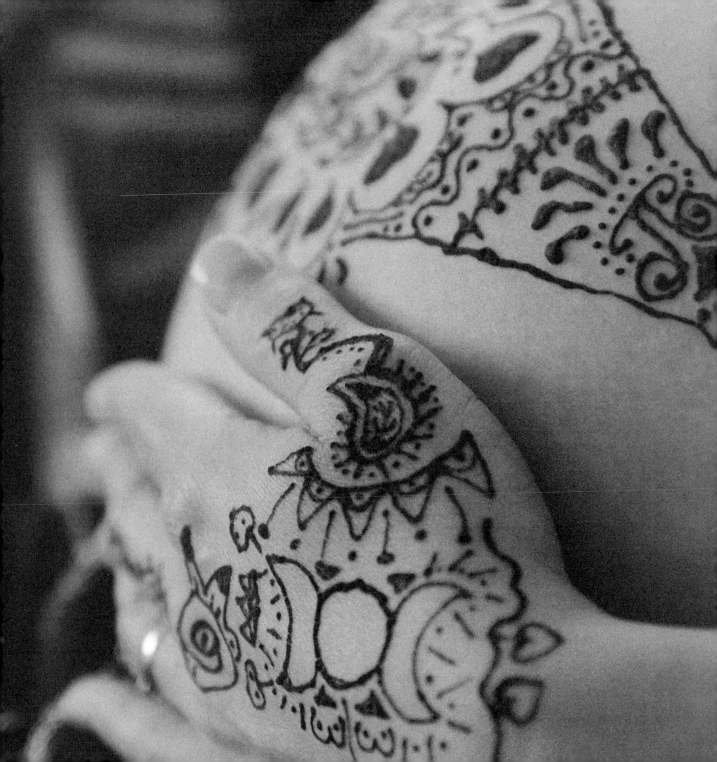

The **circle** is an ancient and universal symbol of community, unity, and feminine power.

BLESSINGWAY CEREMONIES CREATE a sacred and safe environment where a mother-to-be can explore the challenges and joys that lie before her as she approaches birthing and mothering. Surrounded by the most important women in her life, she gains a sense of power, confidence, and support that will help her rise to motherhood.

Birth is a key life passage for women. But modern culture has become preoccupied with the arrival of the baby-to-be and has lost touch with birth's profound impact on the expectant mother. While our most common birth preparations focus on getting women physically ready to give birth, the blessingway ceremony helps a woman to prepare mentally, emotionally, and spiritually for the work of birthing, and it opens her to her instinctive abilities, which will guide her as she steps into the role of mother.

A baby shower is the closest event to a blessingway that women participate in today. It is a wonderful *and* practical occasion—a chance to gather family and friends to share in a celebration for the coming of a new baby, and it is an opportunity to provide the expectant mother (or couple) with many of the items necessary to care for a newborn. A baby shower's primary purpose is focused on the baby that is on the way.

A blessingway is different from a baby shower in essence because it offers us the chance to come together in a spiritual setting and share in a sacred time of reflection, support, and celebration that is focused on the mother-to-be. The gifts that are brought to the expectant mother are offered to raise her energy for labor, provide her with comfort and support, and help her welcome her new baby. The blessingway ceremony's main goals are to honor the mother-to-be and to create a circle of support that will cradle her as she prepares to give birth to and mother her child.

There is no right or wrong way to create a blessingway ritual; however, it is important to include several elements in order to achieve powerful results. We have organized these ritual elements into five distinct stages, forming the foundation for every blessingway we create:

Beginning: Helps us establish the safe and special space that is needed to do the work of the ritual

Shifting: Moves us from individual consciousness into the realm of circle consciousness

Focusing: Centers our attention on the mother-to-be as we honor, pamper, and prepare her for her journey

Completing: Affirms our connection to the important work we have done during the ceremony as well as our connection with one another

Feasting: Brings the work of the ritual into our everyday lives and helps us move from sacred space back to social space

The blessingway rituals presented within *Mother Rising* draw upon the rich traditions of many cultures, having been crafted from the mixed heritage and life experiences of many women. Though initially inspired by the earth-based ways of the Native American culture, these rituals are not intended to represent, nor be executed as, reenactments of a sacred Native American Blessingway ceremony. The word "blessingway" is used conceptually, with due honor and respect, to describe a non-Native ceremony that celebrates a woman's passage into motherhood.

When we create blessingways for each other, we women reach outside of ourselves and weave a web of community: a living breathing web of women who are blessing, teaching, and supporting one another— and as a result, we help to give birth to each other's children.

As women, we receive a great deal by coming together in this way. We can raise energy and strength, or provide comfort and support. We can help one another let go of the past, live fully in the present, and embrace the mystery of the future. We learn to honor each other as well as ourselves, and we tap into the vibrant energy of the collective feminine spirit. By connecting on

this level, we gain the power to deepen our friendships, build our communities, feed our spirits, and perhaps even to revitalize our culture.

On Culture and Childbirth

At one time, it was common for women to gather together to empower and support one another as women who kept the hearth, raised the food, prepared the meals, and reared the children. These women shared food, combined child care, and helped each other when someone became ill.

As common practice, older women helped to prepare the young women for marriage and then for childbirth. They continued to support new mothers for many months after giving birth—by providing food, medicinals, and care for older children and by keeping house. Some cultures today still drop everything to carry out the proper rituals for weddings, births, and funerals as a community—and it is often women who are at the center of the preparations for these events.

Today, our American culture as a whole lacks connection to deep tradition. We are such *diverse* people with such *diverse* practices that we share few common rituals for honoring meaningful life events. As we move from

Pathways to Motherhood

There are many ways to become a mother, and pregnancy is only one of them. Adoption, foster parenting, and marriage (or union) with someone who already has a child are all pathways to motherhood. A blessingway is a beautiful ceremony to hold for any woman who is about to become a mother to another living being.

4

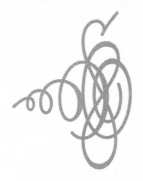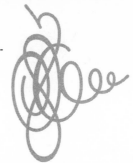

EVERYTHING CONNECTS TO EVERYTHING; THERE-FORE, AS WE CHANGE, THE WORLD CANNOT BUT CHANGE WITH US.

—Marianne Williamson, *Everyday Grace*

one stage of life to the next, many of us discover that we have lost our personal connection to the traditions that once guided us. In addition, the few traditions in which we do participate have become obscured to the point that they have lost their meaning and no longer fulfill their original purpose.

As a result, we've become a culture of individuals who do not understand the value of supporting one another. We have no rituals that serve to carry us through our sometimes difficult life passages.

Living our modern lives, we women often find ourselves giving birth without the personal support of our mothers, our sisters, or our closest friends. We may not live near one another. Some of us are choosing to give birth when we are older—which means that our parents are older, too, and may not be able to be of much help to us.

We can, however, create our own personal communities by bringing into our lives the habit of reaching out to support—and be supported by—those women around us. One way to practice this is by learning to create meaningful rituals.

As women, we really do have a culture of our own, for we hold in common the life peaks of womanhood: childbirth, mothering, and honored elderhood. With respect and care, we can offer opportunities to

one another for deeply felt transformation as we pass through the gateways of our lives.

CHILDBIRTH TODAY

It is a universal truth that if we give something the space to exist, and put our energy into it, then it has a good chance of becoming a reality.

Sadly, we live in a fear-based culture. While pregnant, we train to handle the worst-case scenarios—testing for every possible defect, preparing to heal from tears and cuts that may never happen. We familiarize ourselves with the machinery and the mechanics that will save us or our babies in case something goes wrong.

We learn that birth is a medical emergency, one that we could not possibly handle by ourselves, and that it will take a team of green-swathed surgeons to protect us from the many risks and the imminent harm. Our failure is impending. C-sections are the norm. The baby formula is standing by because we might not have it in us, we alone might not be enough.

A blessingway ritual offers a space for women to release the fears, let go of the worries, and set aside the worst-case scenario training. It creates a positive environment where we can think about the birth process in a different frame of mind. Emphasis is

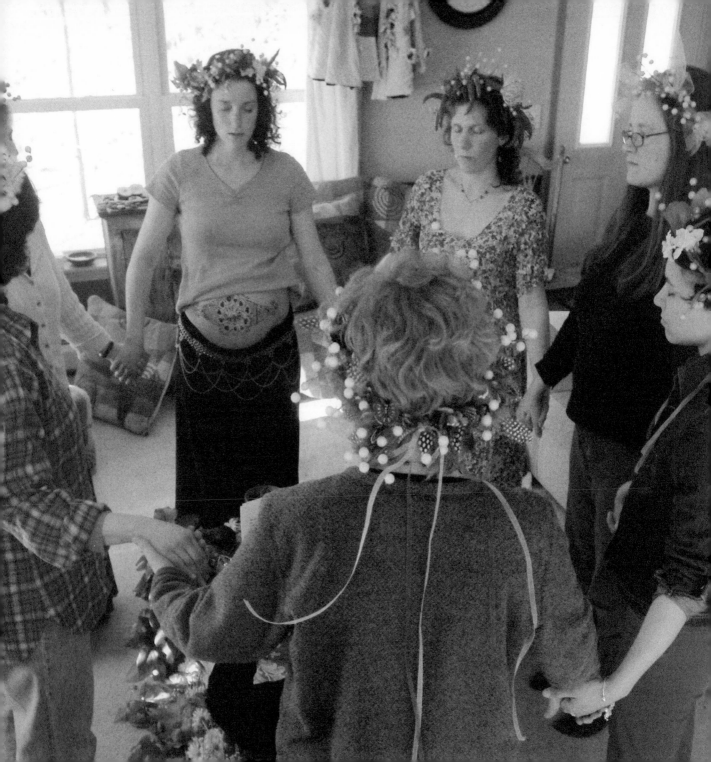

placed on our strengths rather than our inadequacies, and sitting in this place of power, we are affirmed.

During a blessingway ceremony, we get the opportunity to connect to our intuitive selves—the instinctive part of us that hasn't read the books and doesn't know about all the things that might go wrong, the part of us that is simply waiting for the moment when we can finally hold and greet our baby.

By investing some time in the powerful and positive visions of birth as a "blessed event," the reality of it being marvelous begins to grow into being. Cultural habits are strong, so it takes time for new patterns and pathways to emerge. As more women work to create a new vision of birth, one in which we are fully present, the cultural habits around pregnancy and childbirth will eventually shift with us and new traditions will be made.

Women and Ritual

Ritual is what happens when we gather together, with a certain frame of mind and heart, to focus our attention on a specific goal or moment. The main purpose of any ritual is to create conscious connec-

An Altered State of Being

It is interesting to note that the longer we spend together in a blessingway, the stronger our sense of being in an altered state of mind—that odd disassociated feeling of being distanced from what is going on around us—can become. This feeling is a sign that we are relaxing our mind and connecting with our deepest inner self.

When giving birth, we are called upon to let go of our need for physical and mental control and to allow our bodies to widen and spread in order to endure what are sometimes extremes of discomfort and pain for long periods of time. We are then called upon to raise enough power and strength to push our babies out of the dark and narrow spaces of our bodies and into the light of the world. The birthing act requires us both to completely surrender to the experience of labor and to summon amazing personal strength from within. It is through an altered state of being—a relaxed, trusting detachment—that we can indeed find such inner strength.

The wonderful, deep work of a blessingway can introduce an expectant mother to what it is like to move out of her normal mode and into the altered state of consciousness necessary for birth. In this way, the blessingway ritual begins to prepare her for the moment when labor truly does begin.

tion—with ourselves, with others, with the Earth, with Spirit, with God and Goddess. This in turn facilitates our growth, healing, and personal transformation.

Rituals have historically been used to bring meaning to the passages between different stages in life. They make it possible for us to approach any life change or transition with clarity, respect, and awareness by raising our level of attention and participation.

7

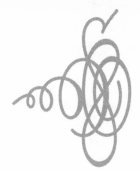
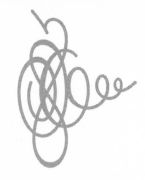

Ritual is about passage, not performance. What matters is that we are willing to participate and remain open to the experience. Through ritual we are reminded that every one of us holds great power within, and when we acknowledge and celebrate this power, we can use it to design our own lives.

Women's rituals help us to explore who we have been, unveil who we are, and celebrate who we're becoming. When we take the time to plan and carry out a ritual, we create a safe space where we can share in intimate detail the things we do not ordinarily speak about in our daily lives. We are able to do this because we pay great attention to creating a sacred and safe environment in which to do our work. In every ritual that takes place, it is important that we are assured that we are safe and well cared for.

The collective energy of a group of women produces a powerful environment. When we come together with a shared intention, we become an amazing force that can effect profound—even miraculous—change.

A group of women can also create an incredibly nurturing environment, for in the company of female people—and all their personal knowledge of what it is to be a woman and live a woman's life—there is a familiarity that makes it easier to open one's self without detailed explanations. Therefore, gatherings of women promote good health and general well-being, which increases our ability to be happy and effective in all areas of our busy lives.

RECLAIMING RITUAL

The word "ritual" is widely used in our culture to signify a focused time for doing things in a familiar way. We often participate in ritual unconsciously, calling it our daily routine. From the time we get ourselves ready for work to the time we put our children to bed, our day is full of little rituals. At holiday times we follow more conscious rituals that we call "traditions." Birthday parties, baby showers, weddings—these events are all rituals.

For those who attend daily or weekly religious gatherings, ritual (along with its root word "rite") is used on a regular basis. Rituals are the various customs that people from all cultures and all walks of life practice to honor significant life events.

We do realize, however, that "ritual" carries negative connotations as well—and herein lies one of our biggest challenges. So we asked ourselves, *"How do we use the word ritual in a way that does not conjure up the image of a spooky gathering?"* (an unfortunate association that pervades our cultural consciousness).

Perhaps, we decided, by doing just this: by reclaiming it—by using the word ritual and reinfusing it with its deepest meaning. As we searched for the perfect words to define ritual, we found that they had already been said by Thomas Moore in his book *The Education of the Heart*: "*Any action that speaks to the soul and to the deep imagination, whether or not it also has practical effects, is ritual.*"

The Power of the Circle

There is great power in sitting in a circle. For when we sit facing one another, we open ourselves to each other, working together instead of working alone. We make trusting connections with one another in our circle and contribute in mutually supportive ways. Doing our work in a circle brings out the very best in each of us.

Working in this way, we open ourselves to the limitlessness of the circle's ability to reenergize and reengage us as our work continues. A perception turns and revolves as we toss it among ourselves, each looking at it from our own perspective. A concept remixes and remakes itself as we share it, shedding pieces that are no longer needed. New and healthier

There's a Little Witch in Every Woman

Feminist, earth-based spirituality plays a very important part in what we are trying to accomplish through our rituals. Because of this, you will find certain practices sprinkled throughout this book that you may have previously associated with witches or witchcraft. What scholars have learned is that many wisewomen, midwives, and healers (women of knowledge, skill, and power in professions over which men wished to assume control) were labeled "witches" in the past. As a tactic to undermine their authority in a patriarchal system, these women were persecuted, their practices forbidden. Consequently, the worth of women was diminished, and the strength of our female lineage was lost. The work of reclaiming our inherent power came into focus only a few decades ago.

We believe that, as women, we owe it to ourselves not to let a word such as "witch" stand in the way of realizing our full potential. We hope that you will keep an open mind as you explore the possibilities and ideas presented in this book, for there is still much to do in the vital, collective process of recovering the wisdom of our past. Recognizing the value and knowledge of our ancestors is central to our coming into our own full power as women.

ideas begin to take shape and come to rest within each of us.

At the very heart of all things that exist, especially at the center of a circle used for ritual, is the Source, however we define it: Spirit, God, Goddess, love, Mother Nature. It is the guiding light of all things, people, and ways. When divine inspiration is unveiled, and therefore actively at work in the center of a circle, there are no limits to the depth and breadth of the work that we can collectively bring about.

When *women* form a circle, we open ourselves to the power of the collective *feminine* spirit—the feminine, creative expression of the Divine—which guides the women's work that we have yet to do. Together, working in our circle, we receive the same guidance that has led great women of all ages to states of divine grace and timeless wisdom.

Under the guidance of the Divine, we rediscover our inherent connection with the sacred, spiritual, feminine power that lives in us and around us. By keeping the center of a circle sacred and attuned to such radiant inspiration, we reinfuse everything that we do as women with the brilliance of the collective feminine spirit's most grace-filled blessings.

How Blessingways Create Community

Women often come to participate in blessingways from different areas of the mother-to-be's life. Sometimes our only connection to each other is through her. But as we travel together through the dynamic, and sometimes intimate, stages of the ritual, we come to know one another quite differently. During a blessingway, we unveil pieces of our true selves as we participate together in supporting the mother-to-be. We are moved and touched by each other. Therefore our relationship with one another changes, and by the end of the blessingway, we are closer.

We begin as a group that is centered on meeting the needs of a woman about whom we all care, perhaps more than ever at that moment. Through the joyful, revealing work of the blessingway, she not only learns that she is supported from within by her own natural abilities, but from without by the women who are circled around her. Together, we guide the mother-to-be so she can ride the waves of childbirth with confidence and strength.

As the mother-to-be finds herself encircled by women who care for her, the other women find amity. The blessingway ritual gives us the opportunity to create a (seemingly) temporary community of women that, in fact, becomes a permanent one. For as we offer our continued support to the mother-to-be beyond the day of the blessingway, we find ourselves also wanting to continue our relationships with one another. Our shared experience of the blessingway brings us much closer together, and we become a circle of friends.

Who Should Use This Book?

Our main goal for creating *Mother Rising* was to inspire and encourage women everywhere to explore the idea of coming together to celebrate and honor a friend's or family member's journey into childbirth and motherhood.

We have worked together for many years to develop a joyful, exciting, and deeply meaningful ceremony that acknowledges, commemorates, and supports this significant and intensely personal time in a woman's life, and wanted to share our experience.

If you are interested in creating a blessingway ceremony for a friend or family member—even if you've never planned (or attended) this kind of event—be assured, you can do it; we will guide you every step of the way. Within this book you will find the elements of a blessingway ritual explained in detail, event planning tips, and many examples, suggestions, and checklists to help get you going.

When we first started to plan blessingways, we read many books and borrowed formats from existing women's rituals. Like us, you will probably grow to develop your own ceremonies that will reflect your personal goals, skills, and beliefs.

Remember, there is no right or wrong way to create a blessingway. Regardless of how simple or elaborate your ritual ends up being, it will be both a beautiful way to welcome a friend or family member into motherhood and a very memorable experience.

A BLESSINGWAY FOR EVERY WOMAN

A blessingway can be held for any woman, whether she is a member of a specific religion, someone who follows her own spiritual path, or someone who claims no faith or spiritual practice at all. It is a ceremony that can be designed to provide a deeply meaningful and transformational experience for a mother-to-be while honoring her personal belief system.

There are many ways that women can connect to the work of a blessingway. Some will make this connection through their sense of self, some through their relationship with God or Spirit, and some through their friendships with other women.

The commonalities of the "spirit of life" far outweigh the differences. Many women will be able to find blessingway elements within this book that express their personal understanding of the world we live in, and as a result, be able to tailor this ceremony to reflect their own individual beliefs and practices.

AN IMPORTANT NOTE FOR MOTHERS-TO-BE

If you are pregnant—or expecting to become a mother by adopting, foster parenting, or marrying someone with a child—and you are interested in having a blessingway, we strongly suggest that you talk to a friend or relative about coordinating and facilitating your ritual. (You can offer them this book as a valuable resource.) They will certainly need to gather input from you to gain a general sense of what you're interested in doing; beyond that, the specifics of the blessingway should really come as somewhat of a surprise to you.

This is important for several reasons:

- The impact of your blessingway will be much greater if you are free to experience the ritual in the moment.
- Becoming too involved in the specific planning, coordination, or facilitation of your blessingway will keep you in your head, instead of in your heart.
- It is an excellent lesson in "letting go."
- To receive a blessingway is to receive a special gift— an experience that has more impact on us when we don't know what lies within the beautiful package.

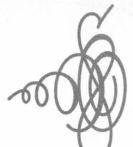
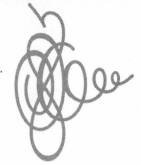

HOW WE WELCOME OUR CHILDREN INTO THE WORLD
REFLECTS OUR HIGHEST HOPES AND DREAMS FOR THEM.

—Carroll Dunham, *Mamatoto: A Celebration of Birth*

AND WHAT ABOUT THE FATHERS-TO-BE?

The information presented in *Mother Rising* is by no means for women's eyes only. The rituals presented here are intended to stimulate and inspire men as well as women. At the same time, being women ourselves, it is not really appropriate for us to speak about how to create a man's pathway to fatherhood. Only men know the real feelings and issues around becoming a father. Only men know what they need to do to process their thoughts and feelings and make this transition.

However, the blessingway ritual's impact on women is so profound that we wholeheartedly encourage men to honor themselves and one another in a similar way. The blessingway concept is not exclusive to women. Many men understand the power of ritual and are weaving it into their lives.

Building a Powerful Blessingway

For more than twenty years now, knowledge of this powerful ritual has been shared between us, woman to woman, circle to circle. Today, many women in our community gather together to create blessingways. Our primary task has remained simple: to raise a mother-to-be's energy and strength that she can carry with her throughout labor and birth and on into the life-changing role of motherhood. Over time our rituals have evolved, reflecting our personal growth as well as our further understanding of the ritual process. As we experiment with the ritual design and alter the pattern of ceremony for each woman we honor, the beauty and power of these events remain inherent.

You'll soon discover that to plan a blessingway is to set off on a great adventure. Now, as you turn the next page, you'll be taking that first step and starting to explore the exciting possibilities!

CHAPTER 2

Planning a
Blessingway

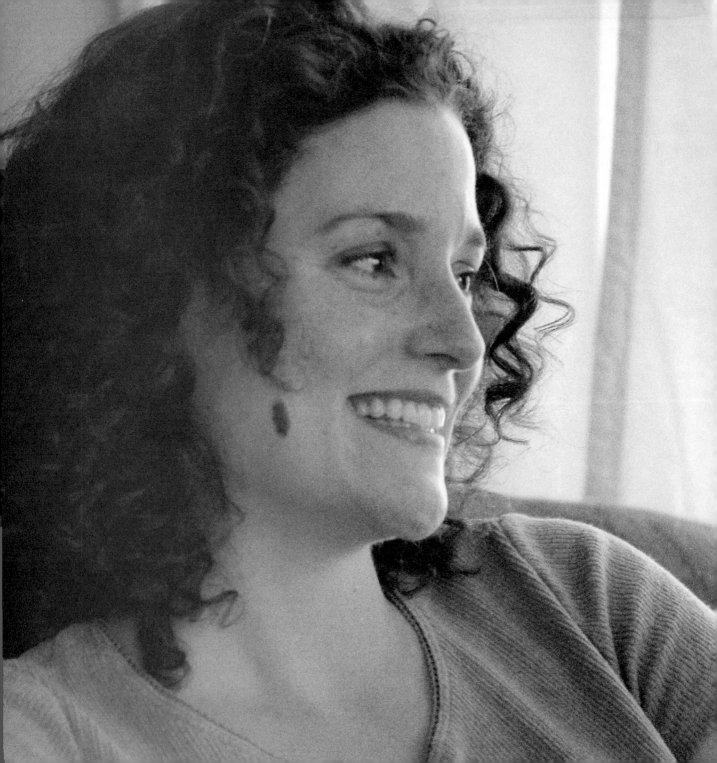

The Maori **Koru** symbolizes new beginnings, life, growth, and harmony.

OUR MODERN LIVES MOVE QUICKLY. For many of us, every twenty-four hours is filled and even overflowing. It doesn't seem to matter whether we are single and without kids, or the mother of seven children. So when we are presented with the idea of planning a blessingway, it's understandable that our first thought may be: *"Where will I find the time?"* If we stay wrapped up in thinking we have too little time, we are bound to feel powerless and even taken for granted amidst our rush to "get it all done."

As women, we are inherently both power-filled and power-full. Each one of us knows on some level that we do have awesome strength at our core. We feel it when we work long hours, then evening comes, and we work some more. We feel it when crisis hits and our family needs us. We feel it when we create something beautiful or bring happiness through our work. When we claim this power and acknowledge the value of what we have to give, we find we can make more power-full choices about how we spend our time.

A blessingway ritual does take time, energy, and effort to create—but it is worth every moment, thought, and drop of perspiration that is put into it. It is a universal principle that when we give, we also receive, and the value of what we stand to receive by coming together and creating this sacred event is beyond measure. When we choose to invest our time in this way, we are choosing to invest in ourselves.

Getting Started

The best place to start the actual blessingway planning process is with the mother-to-be. If she's a good friend or family member, you may have a sense about the kinds of things she likes, which will help guide you when choosing the ritual elements for her blessingway. But what about her fears and concerns? Is there any aspect of childbirth or motherhood that she's worried about or needs support with?

Get together with her over a cup of tea and find out how she's doing both physically and emotionally. Talk with her about her pregnancy, her expectations about her upcoming birth, and her feelings about becoming a mother. Are there any issues from her past or present that are coming up for her? Does she need help sorting through all those thoughts, feelings, and emotions that often come hand-in-hand with pregnancy? Once you have a clear picture of the mother-to-be's attitudes and issues around the arrival of her child, you'll have what you need to design a blessingway ritual that truly meets her needs.

THE ELEMENT OF SURPRISE

Though the blessingway should be developed with her wishes in mind, the mom-to-be should not know exactly what is going to take place during her ritual. In other words, the content of her ritual should be at least partly a surprise. This way her focus will be on the experience, not on her expectations. By relinquishing control of the event, the mother-to-be will be free to surrender herself to the process and allow the blessingway to do its work.

WHEN TO START PLANNING

The blessingway date usually falls somewhere between four and six weeks before the baby is due. To allow you about a month and a half to two months to plan the event, we suggest you begin the blessingway planning process three months before the baby's due date.

Is it imperative that you have this much planning time? Not at all. A very simple blessingway ritual can easily be pulled together in a week, or even in a couple of days. It ultimately will be up to you to determine the amount of time you'll need to plan and organize the type of event you wish to have. (See the appendix for a planning checklist and other helpful information.)

Creating a Guest List

One of a blessingway's primary goals is to create a safe and nurturing environment for the mother-to-be by forming a strong and intimate circle of women. This circle not only serves as the "safe container" in which the mother-to-be will do her work, but it will also be the new mother's support network after her baby is born.

Very often, the women we invite to participate in a blessingway ritual will come from many different relationship circles in the mother-to-be's life—her family circles, her religious or spiritual circles, her parenting circles, her work circles, her recreational circles. The blessingway event itself creates yet another circle: a circle of women, with different relationships not only to the woman who is being honored, but to each other as well. These women may already be intimate with one another, may be casual friends, or may have never met before the day of the blessingway. We may invite women with children, women without children, best friends, fellow playgroup moms, coworkers, and female relatives. No matter what the mix, no matter who we are or where we've come from, time and time again, the experience is this: when women come together for a blessingway, incredible things happen.

There are two ways to create the list of women who will attend; they are as follows:

- The mother-to-be may already have an idea of the women she wants to invite, such as friends and family members whom she feels are important to have there.

- The mother-to-be may want to invite women to her blessingway based on their ability to support the work she needs to do during the ritual.

The most important consideration for the mother-to-be when choosing the guests for her blessingway is

Questions for the Mother-to-Be

Even if you know the expectant mother well, she may hold a few surprises. Take a glance at the list below to be sure that you know where she stands. The answers to these questions will also come in handy when you get further into planning the event:

• How is she feeling physically? Emotionally?

• Where is she having her baby? Who will attend the birth?

• Does she have any concerns about giving birth?

• Does she have any concerns about becoming a mother?

• Will she stay at home or return to work?

• Is her family supportive of her birthing and parenting choices?

• How do her other children feel about the baby?

• What are some of her favorite things to do? (For example, does she dance, sing, or practice yoga?)

• What kind of spiritual practice does she have?

• What kind of music does she like?

• Does she have any allergies or sensitivities to foods, flowers, scents, and so on?

• Where would she like to have her blessingway held?

• Whom would she like to invite?

• Does she feel the potential guests will be able to support her birthing and parenting choices? (This is really important!)

• If she's familiar with blessingways, is there any specific element that she'd like to have included in her ritual?

that she keep in mind her concerns and goals related to her passage into motherhood. Encourage the mother-to-be to invite only those women whom she feels will be able to support her chosen path (natural

birth, water birth, homebirth, and so on). It is imperative that she feels both comfortable and relaxed enough during her blessingway ritual to dive deeply into a place of surrender—a place where she will find the valuable tools that will empower her to birth her baby with confidence.

During a blessingway, women tend to connect on a deeper level than one might initially suspect. Be sure to include the women whom the mother-to-be feels have the capacity to open (and stretch) themselves, and when designing the blessingway (covered in chapters 3 through 8), choose ritual elements that have the potential to touch them deeply. Every woman who attends the blessingway will be changed in some way as a result of the experience.

CONSIDERING A COED BLESSINGWAY?

The mother-to-be will most likely feel more at ease when working in a circle comprised only of women. The more intimate her relationship with these women, the more easily she will be able to explore what is really at stake for her (her hopes and fears, concerns, and expectations) in becoming a mother.

For some couples, however, walking the pathway to parenthood is something that they really want to do together. Coed blessingways are a very different event, as male energy is unlike female energy. By nature, males are more projective and females are more receptive. It's tricky to honor and work with both energies at the same time, though it certainly can be done.

A blessingway ritual that attends to both the soon-to-be father and the mother-to-be will have a different set of goals than a ritual that is focused solely on the mother-to-be, and therefore, will require a different set of ritual elements. For example, it would be important to create activities that honor, affirm, and strengthen the partnership of the parents-to-be in addition to honoring them each as individuals.

Choosing a Location

After you have met with the mother-to-be and gained a rough idea of how many blessingway guests will be invited, you can start thinking about the event location. The best choice is the home of the woman who is being honored, for the energy that will be generated on that day will be tremendous and will linger long after the guests have departed. This remaining supportive energy will be an ongoing gift to the mother-to-be after the blessingway is over. If her house in not an option, choose a location that lends itself to creating the atmosphere you want, while providing the practical amenities you'll need.

The location you *ultimately* choose should have a room or an area that is big enough to comfortably seat the guests (either on the floor or in chairs), as well as enough space to carry out the ritual activities that you have selected for the blessingway (see chapters 3 through 8). Think carefully about the expectant mother's requirements. Pregnant women usually need to eat, drink, and visit the restroom frequently—so be sure you can accommodate these basic needs.

The space you create for a blessingway must be both sacred and safe—a place where the women will feel secure physically as well as emotionally. Privacy is also very important! When holding the ritual in someone's home, other household members should be encouraged to be out of the house on the day of the event. Husbands and boyfriends may enjoy gathering with each other at a different location, or they may opt to take the older children on a special outing to celebrate the upcoming arrival of their new sibling. "Displaced" family members can be invited to return for the feast that follows the blessingway—just be careful of the timing so their return does not interrupt the ritual itself.

Inviting Guests

When inviting guests to the blessingway, you have several opportunities to describe the mother-to-be's upcoming event and to explain what a blessingway is. A save the date card, sent significantly in advance of the event, requests that guests set aside this important date, and a detailed invitation that follows later tells them what to expect and how to prepare. A follow-up phone call is another opportunity to check in with invited guests to confirm who can attend and to ensure that everyone is comfortable participating in the ritual.

SAVE THE DATE CARDS

You'll certainly want to send out invitations to the blessingway, and we'll get to composing those next. For now, help ensure that the carefully chosen guests will be able to attend by sending out a save the date card ahead of time, two months before the event. Unlike the invitations, which will be sent out a month before the event, these advance notice cards will contain only general information. The simple save the date card (or an email) should include the following information:

- Name of the woman for whom the blessingway is being held
- Date of the blessingway (and time frame, if you know it at this point)
- Information about blessingway ceremonies

BLESSINGWAY INVITATIONS

Blessingway invitations should go out one month before the blessingway (or giving as much lead time as possible). After you've read chapters 3 through 8, learning about the five stages of a ritual and creating a rough blessingway outline, you can compose invitations. They will contain all the specific information that guests will need to know, such as what to bring to the gathering, according to the elements and activities you've decided to include in the ritual.

**You are invited to attend
a Blessingway honoring Tanya**
Sunday, April 13, 2003
1:00 p.m. to 5:00 p.m.

———— • ————

A blessingway is a special ceremony designed to acknowledge, honor, and celebrate a woman's journey into motherhood. Different from a baby shower, a blessingway's main goal is to provide a loving place where an expectant mother can explore the challenges and joys that lie before her as she approaches childbirth and motherhood. Surrounded by the most important women in her life, she will gain a sense of power, confidence, and support that will help her before, during, and after the birth of her child.

In your invitations, restate the basic information from the save the date cards, plus provide the details:

- Name of the woman for whom the blessingway is being held
- Date of the blessingway
- Information about blessingway ceremonies
- Time and schedule of events
- List of items to bring (include both gifts and food)
- Location of the blessingway
- Any additional information the guests may need in order to comfortably participate in the ritual elements or activities that have been planned
- Name and number of the RSVP contact person

RSVP OPPORTUNITIES

A blessingway is often a new experience for a guest, so a one-on-one conversation with each woman can help her overcome any fear of the unknown and gain a sense of what to expect. RSVP phone calls create great opportunities to connect with the participants ahead of time, answer their questions, and prepare them practically and spiritually for the blessingway experience.

Here are some things you can go over:

Ritual details: What you will be doing together (in general) and why the event will take as long as you've estimated. Assure them they will have lots of fun, the time will seem to fly by, and that everyone—not just the mom-to-be—will feel great and full of energy afterward!

Gift suggestions: Advise them based on the nature of your ritual outline. (See chapter 6 for gift suggestions.)

Food parameters and potluck coordination: Sometimes expectant (and new) moms can't have spicy foods, or they may be vegetarians. (Check with the mom-to-be ahead of time.)

What to wear: A blessingway is a special occasion, so guests will want to dress their best to celebrate with and honor the mother-to-be. They will also need to bear in mind the overall plan and location of the blessingway when choosing their attire—especially if the circle will be working outside.

Late arrivals and early departures: If a guest will be arriving late or leaving early, ask her ahead of time to be mindful and create as little disruption as possible. Communicate this simply by requesting she "slip in or sneak out" as she comes or goes.

WISHY-WASHY GUESTS

So what do you do if, after you've provided information and answered all her questions, a guest is still noncommittal (or even resistant) about attending? It's tricky, but the best way we have found to address this predicament is by getting together with the mother-to-be to go over any indefinite responses. A choice will generally need to be made—either changing the guest list or altering the ritual—and the mother-to-be should decide what to do. She may ask you to modify the ritual to accommodate certain guests. For instance, if many women are concerned about the length of the blessingway, you might need to simplify your ritual format so it can be accomplished within a shorter period of time.

Occasionally, you may come across someone who feels that the concept of a blessingway is in conflict with her personal belief system. If you experience this, the wisest choice may be to openheartedly support the woman in not attending the blessingway as opposed to attempting to convince her otherwise. It will not be to anyone's benefit if she attends the ritual and sits in discomfort—whether she holds her feelings inside or expresses them openly.

Distributing Responsibilities

For very simple blessingways, one or two women can easily assume all the different roles and responsibilities necessary to organizing and leading the ritual. How-

Coordinating Post-Blessingway Meals

Assign someone to coordinate and keep track of any post partum meal deliveries pledged to the mother-to-be. This woman will need to touch base with the new mother to create a schedule that meets her needs. The meal coordinator should discuss the following with the new mom:

• When would she like her meals to start being delivered?
• How often would she like to have meals delivered? (Two or three meals per week is average.)
• What time would she like her meals delivered by?
• Are frozen meals okay? Does she have freezer space?
• Does she (or anyone in her family) have any food restrictions, allergies, or preferences (for example, vegetarian, no dairy, or non-spicy foods), or is it anything goes?

The meal coordinator should follow up and remind each woman when her date is coming up, and then verify that each meal was, in fact, delivered. For those women who aren't into cooking, suggest they deliver take-out or pre-prepared foods. If time is a factor that precludes personal delivery, giving a gift certificate for a take-out meal will also be appreciated. A new mom will often have her hands full, so stocking her freezer with prepared frozen meals or her cupboards with granola and trail mix can be a great help.

One person should, however, take on the role of primary blessingway facilitator and oversee all aspects of the ritual, including planning, designing, and leading the blessingway.

As part of the planning process, consider assigning coordinators to take care of the invitations, music, food, supplies, and post-blessingway follow-up tasks. Find someone (who is not involved in leading the ritual) to take photos during the event. Videotaping may also be an option; however, this can create confidentiality issues, so check with all the guests (as well as the mother-to-be) to determine whether or not this is appropriate. Don't forget to enlist help for setup and cleanup on the day of the blessingway.

POST-BLESSINGWAY SUPPORT

Your support of the mother-to-be should not end on the day of the ritual. In addition to delegating tasks specific to the blessingway event, ask a member of your planning team to check in frequently with the mother-to-be after the blessingway to ensure

ever, if the blessingway you're planning contains a wide variety of ritual elements, you'll want to involve as many women as possible in the preparations. that her energy remains high and to assess her need for additional support (see chapter 10 for what you can do to help her).

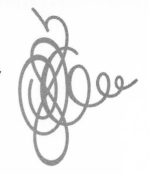

[A WOMAN'S] NEED FOR ATTENTION AND AN UNDER-
STANDING EAR DOES NOT DISAPPEAR WHEN THE BABY
APPEARS. IT INCREASES DRAMATICALLY.

—Jennifer Louden, *The Pregnant Woman's Comfort Book*

Make sure that someone will be coordinating any postpartum gifts of service offered to the mother-to-be, such as prepared meals (you'll read about gifts in chapter 6). Meal coordination is especially important because a new mom will not have time to schedule meal deliveries, nor should she ever have to scramble to feed her family if a promised dinner doesn't show up!

PHONE TREES AND LABOR CANDLES

After the blessingway, the ritual participants will want to be apprised of any new developments in the mother-to-be's journey, such as when she goes into labor, when her baby has been born, or when she gets "the call" from the adoption agency. The best way to update everyone is by using a phone tree. A phone tree is a list made up of each guest's name and phone number, as well as any additional friends or relatives whom the mother-to-be would like notified. Each individual on the list is responsible for calling the person listed after them on the phone tree, which means everyone will be responsible for making only one phone call—unless they can't reach the person they call. (If this happens, they should leave a message, then move down the list and continue on until they speak directly with someone.) Plan to create the phone tree in advance, and be sure to make enough copies to hand out to all participants before they leave the blessingway event.

To further strengthen the circle's support of the mother-to-be, consider making a basket of votive candles available to guests after the blessingway. Invite the women to take home a candle to light in support of the mother-to-be when they learn that she has gone into labor, or that she has left to get the child she is adopting.

CHAPTER 3

Designing Your Ritual

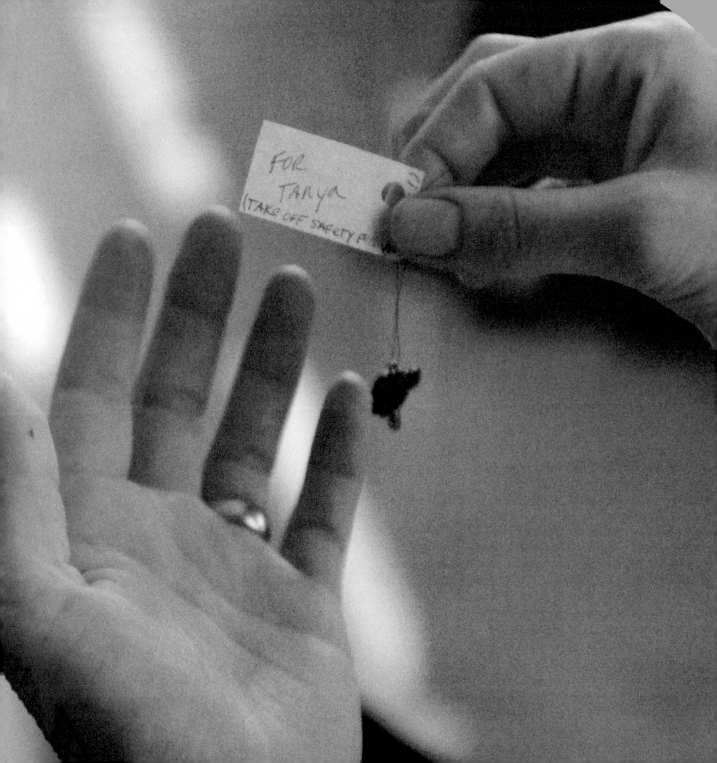

Sesa Woruban is a West African Adinkra symbol that means
"I transform my life."

IF CREATING A BLESSINGWAY RITUAL seems at all daunting to you right now, try planning a ritual that is very simple, rather than abandoning the entire concept. A blessingway doesn't need to be an over-complicated undertaking.

Or perhaps you're thinking this stuff is all too hippy-dippy for you. Well then, stay in your comfort zone and don't design a "way out there" event. No matter how you put a blessingway together, it will be an amazing experience.

The Five Stages of a Ritual

Soon you will learn all you need to know about the five stages of a ritual (discussed in chapters 4 through 8). It's important to familiarize yourself with this information before you start designing your blessingway, so before you get into all the details, take a look at the following overview of what actually happens during each stage:

STAGE 1 Beginning: We create a ritual space that looks and feels special. Guests need to become centered and ready to participate in a sacred ceremony. We form a circle to create a container of support for the mother-to-be. When we call in the presence of the Divine, we're asking for all the help we can get.

STAGE 2 Shifting: We state the blessingway's purpose so we all know what we're doing and why we're doing it, and while we're at it, we share our intention with the powers that be. Introducing ourselves helps us connect with one another. We help the mother-to-be let go of any negative beliefs or fears she may be carrying so that she can embrace all the blessings, prayers, and honor we wish to bestow upon her.

STAGE 3 Focusing: We honor, pamper, and adorn the mother-to-be to fill her with positive and em-powering energies. We tell her stories to encourage her, offer blessings to support her, and give her gifts that will help guide her on her journey.

STAGE 4 Completing: Having invested so much time and energy in preparing the mother-to-be, we ensure that the divine forces have, in fact, heard our requests for her safe passage. We raise energy to affirm and charge the work we've done and to send our good intentions out into the world. We weave a web to maintain our connection with one another beyond the day of the ritual. When our work is done, we thank and release the divine powers we've invited to join us and open our circle so we may move on to the final stage of our ritual.

STAGE 5 Feasting: We end our ritual by sharing food together in celebration. We eat together to ground our energy, help us shift from sacred space back to social space, and bring the work of the ritual into our everyday lives.

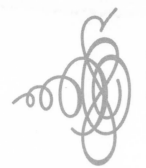
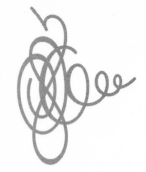

Creating an Outline

Now that you're more familiar with the stages of a ritual, find a notepad and pen and start reading chapters 4 through 8 carefully, noting the specific elements that look especially meaningful or fun to you. You will quickly discover that there are many ways to accomplish each ritual element, so remember that you need only choose one technique or method, not several. For example, for cleansing and purification, you may choose to use a smudge stick or water, but not both. Keep the mother-to-be's objectives in mind to ensure that you're choosing activities that she'll enjoy or will address her needs.

Consider working in a break during your ritual. Even though the women in the circle are welcome to take care of their needs at any time during the blessingway, this assures a pause for everyone. A good place to initially schedule a break is between the shifting stage, when you release fears, and the focusing stage, when you honor the mother-to-be. However, when leading the ritual, you may find you need to take the break at a different time if the group's energy requires it sooner or it would be better saved for later.

When we first started creating blessingways, we clung to our ritual outlines—in their entirety, not just break times—and

Blessingway Themes

A strong guiding principle in the ritual design process is the emergence of a theme. This theme will most likely come forth from the information you gathered when talking to the mother-to-be. Take care to really listen to the mother-to-be's desires and concerns; determining a blessingway theme will then help you to select the ritual elements that best address her needs. Theme's we've designed rituals around include:

• Bonding with the new baby
• Developing a successful nursing relationship
• Having the first boy child in the family
• Achieving a successful VBAC (Vaginal Birth after Cesarean)
• Creating family unity
• Maintaining a close bond with an older child

A Blessingway for Shawna

Shawna's ritual followed a simple format and took about three hours to complete with a circle of ten women. (To see more ritual outline examples, go to www.blessingwaybook.com.) This is a great introductory blessingway outline:

- Welcome and Introductions
- Casting the Circle: A Clarity Prayer
- Stating the Purpose
- Meditation: "Waves: A Birth Visualization" by Carl Jones
- Summoning the Four Directions
- Introducing Goddesses
- Summoning Demeter
- Sharing Altar Items
- Releasing Fears
- Break

- Honoring and Pampering Shawna (hair brushing, herbal footbath, shoulder massage)
- Presenting Gifts
1. A gift that symbolizes the power of relaxation, strength, or healing
2. Beads for Shawna's birth bracelet, the baby's bracelet, and for Iris's bracelet to honor her new role as big sister

3. A creative postpartum gift
- Candle Blessing
- Weaving a Web
- Releasing the Four Directions and the Goddess Demeter
- Closing: An African Prayer
- Opening the Circle
- Feast

were thrown off when things didn't proceed according to plan. Don't do that. When the time comes, use your ritual outline as a guide rather than a script. There will be times when it is necessary to change or let go of scheduled ritual elements that just don't fit in the moment. A blessingway doesn't have to flow in the exact order of your outline to produce powerful results. If you take care not to pack too much into your ritual outline, it will be easier to make adjust-

ments when necessary during the actual blessingway.

After you've generated your initial list of ritual possibilities, you can form the first draft of your blessingway outline. Now is a good time to take a moment and thumb through the checklists and information we've provided at the back of the book (see the appendix on page 117). These tools will be especially helpful if you've never designed a blessingway ritual before.

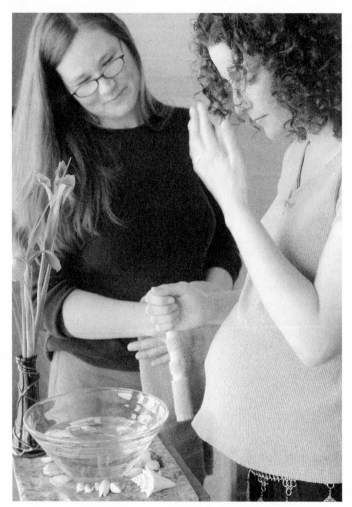

how you can involve others (in addition to the primary facilitator) in various segments of the ritual. Invited guests may express an interest in leading a certain activity, but if not, consider the skills and talents the participants have to offer. You can approach potential leaders ahead of time, or simply invite them in the moment to read a passage or to guide the circle through a particular element.

The Dynamic Nature of Ritual Elements

Even though we have organized each basic ritual element into one of five stages (as seen in chapters 4 through 8), this doesn't mean that an element can't be incorporated into a different stage. Some ritual elements, such as connecting through meditation, can be used to carry out a variety of ritual goals. For example, meditation works equally well as a way of centering each individual, cleansing and purifying the women, casting the circle, opening to the Divine, and raising or grounding energy.

Certain elements, such as readings, make wonderful introductions to blessingway segments, moving the circle of women from one stage to the next or helping us to shift into a certain frame of mind. There are many stories to tell: stories about women coming together, stories about

The more women who are involved in the ritual process, the richer the ceremony becomes. So while you're working on your outline, start thinking about

birth, stories about bonds between mother and child.

Activities such as singing and dancing can be woven into any stage of a ritual to effectively set the mood or the tone for the work ahead. Playing mindfully chosen recorded music will also achieve this, as well as serve to anchor guests to the blessingway event long after the ritual is over. Whenever participants hear a song or piece of music from the blessingway, they will receive a powerful reminder that reconnects them to the work of the ritual. Incorporating music and movement into your blessingway will raise the energy of the group and enhance the overall experience, so go for it! (See page 137 for music suggestions.)

Chants We Love

These traditional chants are both beautiful and powerful when included in a blessingway:

Chants for Casting a Circle
"River of Birds"
"Earth My Body"

Chants for Calling the Divine
"Grandmother Song"
"Isis, Astarte, Diana"

Chants for Connecting
"Ancient Mother"
"Mother I Feel You"
"We All Come from the Goddess"
"Place of Power" (by Anne Hill)

Chants for Weaving a Web
"Spiraling into the Center"
"We Are the Flow"

Chants for Releasing
"Rise with the Fire"
"Fire, Fire, Fire" (by Cynthia R. Crossen)

Chants for Raising Energy
"Wearing My Long Wing Feathers"
"We Are a Circle"

Chants for Opening a Circle
"We Are a Circle within a Circle"
"May the Circle Be Open"
"May the Long Time Sun"

(See page 137 for songbooks containing these and other wonderful chants.)

The Element of Time

The amount of time that it takes to carry out a ritual varies dramatically. Some blessingways last a couple of hours while others last the whole day. It's best to plan a ceremony that is free from time constraints, so the ritual may simply unfold in whatever way it needs to on the day of the event. If this is not possible, expect the gathering to last anywhere from three to six hours, depending upon the number of guests and ritual elements you have included.

Do not be surprised to find, after you've determined the time for your initial ritual outline, that you've planned a two-day event! First drafts often

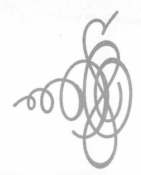

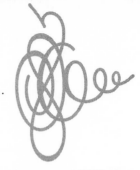

CHANTING OPENS THE INNER EYE OF THE HEART.
IT CLEANS THE MIRROR OF THE HEART SO IT CAN
CLEARLY REFLECT WHAT IS ALREADY INSIDE OF US.

—Krishna Das, *devotional musician*

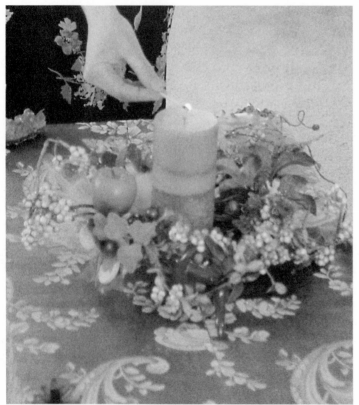

run well beyond a realistic time frame. The next step is to review your outline and start prioritizing, then paring down, taking care not to include too many ritual elements. The ritual facilitator's job will be much easier, and the ritual will flow more naturally, if she is not constantly watching the clock and trying to move people along.

(For more help with estimating time, go to www.blessingwaybook.com.)

CHAPTER 4

Ritual Stage I: Beginning

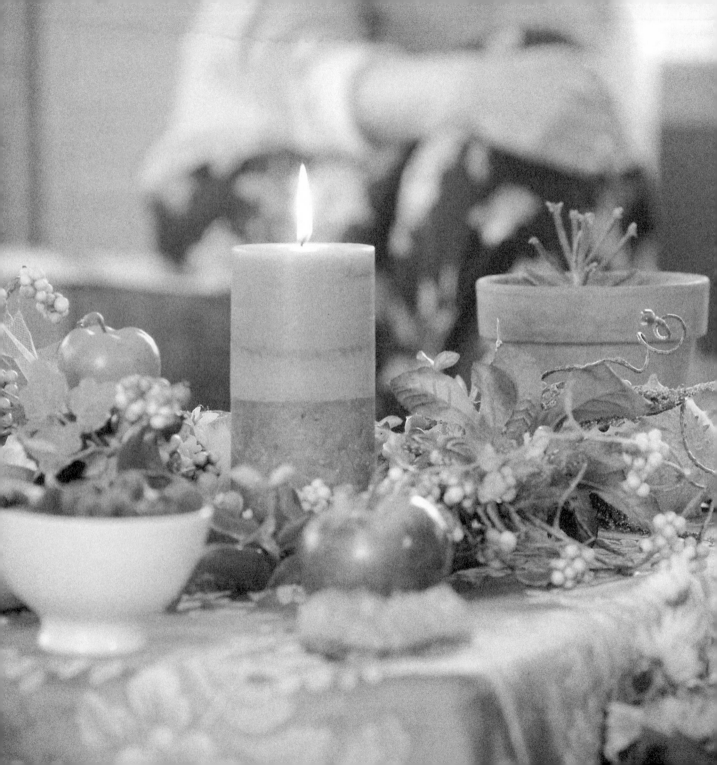

The Native American **Medicine Wheel**, or **Wheel of Life**,
symbolizes all creation.

DURING THE BEGINNING STAGE of a ritual, we need to create a sacred space, a safe container in which to do our ritual work. The elements included in this section accomplish this, plus help us gather and center ourselves, so we will be ready to focus on the work ahead.

Ritual is, in itself, an act of consciously opening ourselves to the presence of Spirit—the Spirit within us, God, universal energy—and it is during the beginning stage that we first make this connection.

Welcome and Overview

Many cultures have traditionally used rituals to bring power and meaning to the passages between different stages in a person's life. Our culture has not, however, commonly used rituals, so the practice of ritual is often new to many women. One way to address blessingway participants' comfort level is by welcoming the guests to the ritual and offering a very general overview of what you'll be experiencing together. Encourage eyeryone to take care of personal needs, such as visiting the bathroom, getting something to drink, or attending to their babies, at any time during the ritual.

Provide the participants with guidelines regarding their involvement in the ritual. Though no one is expected to "perform" during a blessingway, everyone is asked to participate. Participation means that everyone stays attentive, mindful, respectful, aware, and reverent throughout the ritual. It's important to assure guests during this time (and again later on) that a blessingway is a "no fault" ritual; it will help them feel more at ease when you let them know that if they make a "mistake" (like trip or misread something aloud), it's really okay. You don't want anyone to feel nervous or become preoccupied with wondering whether they are "doing it the right way."

A "no fault" ritual is not, however, an "anything goes" ritual. Which is to say that the term "no fault" should not be used to excuse behavior that is inappropriate—thoughtless, disrespectful, or irreverent—nor should it be used to make light of a lack of preparation on the part of the facilitators.

There are other guidelines, or "ritual ground rules," to share with participants at this time as well. In order to create and maintain a nurturing and safe atmosphere, confidentiality is key. This means that what is said in the circle during the course of the ritual needs to remain in the circle. It is vitally important that each woman (not just the mother-to-be) feels safe and secure, so she may share deeply during the ritual

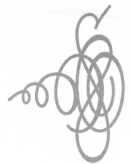

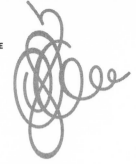

THE WOMEN ARE SILENT, USING THE SMOKE AND THE
PROCESS [TO] LET GO OF OUTSIDE CONCERNS AND
WORRIES TO ENTER FULLY INTO THE RITUAL.

—Diane Stein, *Casting the Circle*

without the fear of others finding out information she may not wish publicized.

Another important point to bring to the group's attention is that a blessingway has the power to evoke very deep emotions. Should the mother-to-be (or anyone in the circle) become emotional, make it clear that no one should touch her, nor offer a tissue to her, unless she asks for it. Though well-intended, these offerings of comfort may actually shut down a wonderful release process.

Finish your overview on a positive note so the group is excited, energized, and can hardly wait to be cleansed, purified, and made ready to experience the wonderful work and fun of the blessingway!

Cleansing and Purification

Cleansing and purification help to turn everyone's attention away from where they were (arranging for child care, preparing gifts and a dish to share, difficulties in their personal lives, and so on) and shift participants' focus to the gathering itself. By allowing their concerns to fall away, participants reveal their most openhearted, centered selves—which frees all the women to become fully present to the ritual experience. Here are three cleansing methods to use at the

beginning of a blessingway, before actually forming the circle, and before inviting guests to be seated.

SMUDGING

Many cultures use various dried herbs or incense to produce a pungent-smelling smoke that is used to cleanse (or smudge) a room, or as a tool to help center people by purifying them physically, spiritually, and emotionally—carrying any unwanted energy, emotions, or distractions up into the ether where it can be transformed.

The dried herbs or incense can be either placed in a bowl loosely or bundled together for burning. Many people like to use a sage bundle (also called a smudge stick) for smudging. Once lit, the sage is allowed to burn until it glows red, then is blown out and allowed to smoke. The smudge stick can be gently waved about, blown on, or fanned with a feather to direct the smoke where it is wanted.

Burning sage is very strong smelling, so before you choose this method of cleansing, find out whether anyone attending the ritual is particularly sensitive to smell. You should also check with the woman hosting the ritual (usually the mother-to-be) to make sure that it will be all right to use smudge within her home.

A good way to coordinate this activity is by guiding the guests to line up from eldest to youngest outside the entrance to the ritual space. Have each woman enter (or reenter) the ritual space after being cleansed and purified by the smudge. (If this needs to occur outside the house, smudge each woman before she comes back into the house, and re-form the line near the entrance to the ritual space.)

Begin the process of smudging by holding the incense or smudge stick near to the participant and then passing the smoke (by fanning it with your hand or a feather) over and around the participant's body. Smudge (smoke) the fragrance over the front and back of each woman, making sure to include her head, hands, and feet. One woman will often agree to smudge the others, and while smudging she may softly say, *"Take a deep breath. Relax, and let the smoke from the burning sage carry away all that is not needed here today."* After being smudged, each woman can then step into the ritual space and take her place in the circle. (You may invite the guests to choose their own seats before the ritual begins, or guide them at this time to be seated in accor-

dance with a preconceived plan.) The woman who has smudged the others may smudge herself or ask to be smudged by another participant when she has finished purifying the line of women. Alternatively, each woman in the circle can smudge herself, holding this same clearing thought in mind while fanning herself

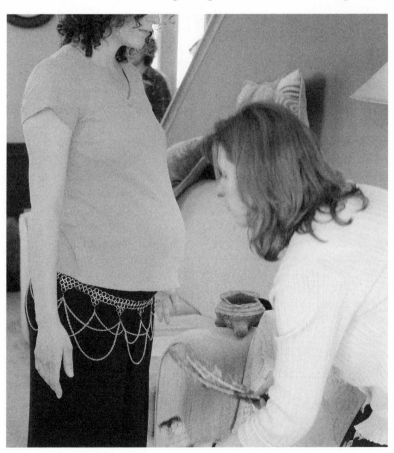

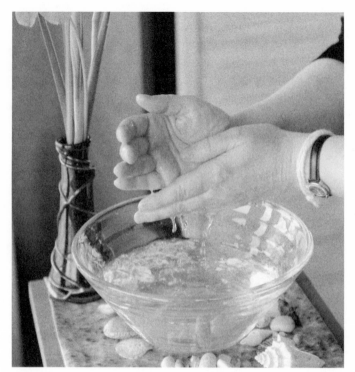

of the ritual space. Ask each guest to dip her hands into the water and release any thoughts, memories, or energies that she does not wish to take with her into the circle. When finished, she may be invited to enter the ritual space and take her place in the circle. Participants should remain standing until everyone has entered the ritual space and the next element of the ritual, casting the circle, has been carried out.

SALT WATER PURIFICATION

Sea salt dissolved into a bowl of spring water can be sprinkled around a room and on each woman with the intention of clearing away old memories and energies related to whatever was present in the room or within the guests before the ritual gathering. When you do this as a group, saying a few intention-setting words while you sprinkle the salt water is a great way to focus the energy of those who are with you. Together and aloud, the women may repeat *"May these waters from the West renew and ready this space for the important work we will do here today."* Once the ritual space has been cleansed, each woman can sprinkle a few drops of salt water on herself, silently let go of the thoughts and energies she doesn't need to bring to the ritual, enter the sacred space, and take her place in the circle. As with the other purification methods, the participants should remain standing until the next task of casting the circle has been completed.

with the smoke. When she is finished, she may pass the smudge stick to the next youngest woman in the line, step into the ritual space, and take her place in the circle. No matter which smudging method you choose, everyone should remain standing throughout the process, and until the circle has been cast (the next element of a ritual).

ROSE WATER PURIFICATION

A bowl of spring water sprinkled with fresh rose petals can be placed in a powder room or just outside

Casting the Circle

When you cast a circle, you are forming a virtual container. The circle is the secure and confidential space you create to welcome women to the ritual experience and allow them to open to their understanding of God or Spirit. Once the purified women form this circle, you lead them to act with reverence, and the work that is done is sacred. When your circle is cast, it is considered "closed," and participants are safe within its confines. There are two ways to cast a circle, by saying a prayer together or by physically defining the circle.

SAY A PRAYER

A prayer, such as the following slight adaptation of the "Prayer for Clarity" from Shea Darian's beautiful book *Seven Times the Sun,* can be used to cast a circle.

Holding hands and becoming still, lead the women to say together: *"Let us form this circle with clear thoughts, wise words, and kind hearts."* There are movements that go along with this particular prayer. If desired, guide the guests to touch their foreheads on "clear thoughts," touch their lips on "wise words," and place a palm over their hearts on "kind hearts," as you recite the prayer together. When the prayer is completed, announce that the circle has been cast, and invite the women to be seated.

PHYSICALLY DEFINE THE CIRCLE

You may choose to cast a circle by defining your ritual space. To do this, carry a lit smudge stick or sprinkle salt water while moving clockwise around the circle (just outside of the circle of women). When you are back at your starting point, announce that the circle has been cast, and invite the participants to be seated.

Opening to the Divine

Opening to the Divine is one of the first things you'll do together as a circle of women. It sets the tone for your special time together. Connecting to a sense of God or Spirit—whatever "the Divine" means to everyone—enables the women to deepen the work they will do for the rest of the day. Think of this segment as a time of prayer that directs the hearts and minds of the women to the sacred nature of blessing-way ritual.

Both inward connection and outward connection to God or Spirit can exist simultaneously. However, because individual perceptions and beliefs vary so greatly, you may find that you need to differentiate between invocation and evocation.

Invocation is the act of calling to mind (heart, body, and soul) certain attributes that exist outside ourselves, and then opening up to the possibility of these things coming to exist within us in the moment of invocation. For some women, an invocation is simply a reminder of the oneness of God or Spirit, a reminder that there is no separation between ourselves and the attributes offered to us by the Divine.

Evocation is the act of calling on the Divine to be present with (or to watch over) us as we work. Evocations may also be used to invite the "spiritual presence" of friends and family members who could not

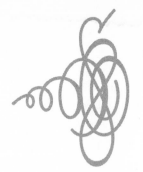
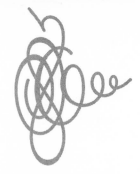

be physically present for the ritual, and to recognize small children who will soon become big brothers or big sisters, so they too may be honored during the blessingway ritual.

It's important to reflect the mother-to-be's understanding of the Divine (as well as her guests', when possible) in the choices you make when designing a ritual. If she does not consider herself to be religious or spiritual, there are many other powerful ways to help her open to the work of the blessingway. Consider using the memory of an inspiring ancestor to help her access her highest and most creative inner knowing. Try guiding her to connect with the women of her blessingway circle, her family, or her community at large—and to gain support through their collective wisdom, strength, spirit, and love—as another powerful way to bring her fully into the work of the ritual.

WORKING WITH THE FOUR DIRECTIONS (OR FOUR QUARTERS)

Since the blessingway is rooted in earth-based traditions, consider summoning the four directions (East, South, West, and North) as part of your ritual. The directions hold powerful, guiding, and protective energies, and when called upon, their qualities awaken parts of our inner selves and bring forth the highest and best we each have to offer to the circle.

The four directions are an essential part of the Native American Medicine Wheel and the Wiccan Magick Circle. You may choose to work with the four directions in your own way, or by following these earth-based practices and their associations between each cardinal direction and a corresponding element of nature, color, and season.

Elemental, Color, and Season Correspondence

Though Native American and Wiccan traditions vary, the following elemental, color, and season correspondence reflects the majority view.

NATIVE AMERICAN TRADITION

East: fire, yellow, spring
South: earth, red, summer
West: water, black, autumn
North: air, white, winter

WICCAN TRADITION

East: air, yellow, spring
South: fire, red, summer
West: water, blue, autumn
North: earth, green, winter

38

Qualities of the Four Directions

The four directions can be thought of as spirits in themselves, each bringing unique gifts such as illumination, adventure, gentleness, and wisdom to the circle. Please note that the elemental associations below follow the Wiccan view.

East: East is associated with air. It is the spirit of balance, greatness, and humility. The East brings the gifts of illumination and great vision. It is the time of spring and new life. The sometimes gentle, sometimes strong winds of the East reveal the way of love, and thus creation, to the circle.

South: South is represented by fire. It encompasses passion, adventure, and discovery. The South offers the lessons of humor, innocence, trust, and appreciation. It is the time of summer and harvest. The South teaches the circle how to walk with courage and fiery determination in the way of growth and balance.

West: West is united with water. It offers us gracefulness, gentleness, honesty, adaptability, and calmness. The westerly water's soothing presence allows peace to fill our hearts. The West guides us to places of great depths that are hard to define. It is the time of autumn and maturity. In appealing to the West, the circle discovers all that life has to offer, and what it takes for us to be all we can be.

North: North is symbolized by earth, solid and sturdy. It is the essence of wisdom, truth, and unfolding trust and wonder. The North brings us to the land of surrender and to quiet, rejuvenating places. It is the time of winter and the ancestors. It gives the circle strength; it is sacred ground, firm under our feet.

Creating Altars for the Four Directions

You'll want to create a separate altar for each direction to contain items symbolic of that direction and the energies or attributes associated with its corresponding element. Set these altars up outside or as part of the circle, positioned in the location of the corresponding direction (which means that someone will need to determine which way is which—East, South, West, and North—before you begin setting up). Your altars should be built on tables if you plan to seat the participants in chairs, or on the floor if everyone will be seated on the ground.

Never created an altar before? Sure you have, just take a look around your home—at all the flat surfaces. If you're like us, many of your end tables, desks, dressers, and mantels are covered with an array of items that include candles, pictures of relatives, and a variety of other treasures that have meaning to you— a shell, a box, a bell, a bowl. Each one of these things is actually a symbol of something much larger (such as beauty, joy, wisdom, or love), and just by looking at these items, we can connect to what they truly stand for—just like when we see an altar in a sacred setting.

To get started on building your four altars, you'll need a few basic items such as altar tables (if using), tablecloths (or altar cloths), and vases of fresh flowers. You'll also want to include a candle on each altar in the appropriate corresponding color. To complete your altars, add a few small objects that represent the qualities of each particular direction. We offer many suggestions below, but keep in mind that the most beautiful altars are often very simple. (See the appen-

39

dix to learn more about the symbolic qualities of everyday objects.)

East altar: Air symbols may include an empty bowl (containing air), bells, chimes, feathers, eggs, fans, incense, pinwheels, kites, books, musical instruments, and images or objects in the form of the sky, birds, dragonflies, or butterflies. Season: spring. Candle color: yellow.

South altar: Fire symbols may include lit candles, chile peppers, hot sauce or salsa, and images or objects in the form of the sun, lions, dragons, coyotes, lizards, geckos, or armadillos. Season: summer. Candle color: red.

West altar: Water symbols may include a bowl of water, shells, sand, water-smoothed stones or sea glass, seaweed, driftwood, pitchers, cups, a lachrymatory (a vial that holds tears), and images or objects in the form of the ocean, mermaids, fish, sea creatures, dolphins, whales, salmon, starfish, sand dollars, black bears, or ravens. Season: autumn. Candle color: black or blue.

North altar: Earth symbols may include a bowl of dirt, rocks, crystals, minerals, salt, stones, metals, mother earth images, plants, flowers, leaves, trees, food, grains, fruits, vegetables, and images or objects in the form of large land animals, bears, white owls, or turtles. Season: winter. Candle color: white or green.

Calling the Four Directions

Here are three scripts for summoning the four directions at the beginning of your ritual—each with a unique focus. Have all circle participants turn to face each direction as it is called. Begin with the East, then call the South, the West, and finally the North. Light the appropriate altar candle after summoning each direction.

BIRTH-INSPIRED SUMMONS: "We welcome the spirit of the **East**, who brings the breath of new life and gives relief from difficult laboring energy. Please be with us today. We welcome the spirit of the **South**, who inspires fiery determination and prompts a baby's first cry. Please be with us today. We welcome the spirit of the **West**, who calms the waters of a baby's uterine home and ensures the plentiful breast. Please be with us today. We welcome the spirit of the **North**, who comes from the land of quiet rejuvenating spaces to tell tales of surrender and of our ancestors. Please be with us today."

ELEMENT-INSPIRED SUMMONS: "Blessed be this gathering with the gifts of the **East**: communication of the heart, mind, and body; fresh beginnings with each rising of the sun; the knowledge of the growth found in sharing silences. Blessed be this gathering with the gifts of the **South**: warmth of hearth and home; the heat of the heart's passion; the light to illuminate the darkest of times. Blessed be this gathering with the gifts of the **West**: the lake's deep commitments; the river's swift excitement; the sea's breadth of knowing. Blessed be this gathering with the gifts of the **North**: firm foundation on which to build; fertile fields to enrich our lives; a stable home to which we may always return."

CIRCLE-INSPIRED SUMMONS: "We beckon to the **East**, bringer of first light. Send your driving winds to carry away from this circle what does not belong here. Open this place for the communion of heart, mind, and soul that is your promise with each new rising of the sun. And to the **South**, whose power is the sun, high in the sky. Cleansing fire, burn away what has no place here. Make way for this circle's heart to become its hearth so our passions are free to grow and glow bright here within it. And to the **West**, governor of the all-encompassing sea. Wash clean this circle to make way for our dreams and feelings to flow freely, so we may find rich and fertile ground upon which to grow. And to the **North**, teacher of surrender, death, change, and of the dark place of womb time. Release what holds us back from becoming vessels for your wintry white purity, and make this circle a firm foundation upon which to stand and to build today."

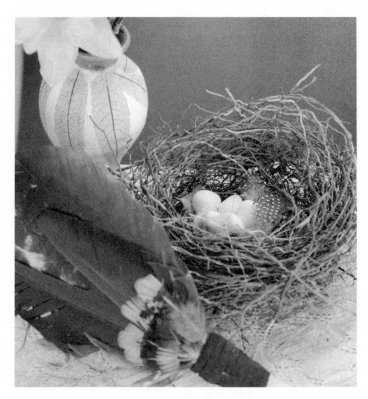

Releasing the Four Directions

When it is time, the four directions are released in reverse order of the way in which they were summoned. Again, all circle participants should turn to face the direction that is being addressed. Begin in the North, then release the West, the South, and finally the East, thanking each direction for what it gave to the circle. Snuff the appropriate altar candle after releasing each direction.

BIRTH-INSPIRED RELEASE: "Spirit of the **North**, we thank you for your presence. You are free to leave our circle. Please remain with (name of the mother-to-be) to give her the ability to surrender to her changing role as she births her baby. Spirit of the **West**, we thank you for your presence. You are free to leave our circle. Please remain with (name of the mother-to-be) to facilitate her rapid physical healing after the birth of her child. Spirit of the **South**, we thank you for your presence. You are free to leave our circle. Please

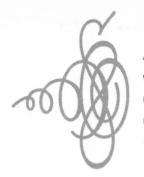
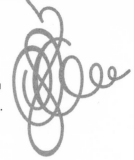

AS WOMEN, WE KNOW [THE GODDESS] BECAUSE
WE ARE SHE. EACH WOMAN, NO MATTER HOW
POWERLESS SHE MIGHT FEEL, IS A CELL WITHIN
HER VAST FORM, AN EMBODIMENT OF HER ESSENCE.

—Jalaja Bonheim, *Aphrodite's Daughters*

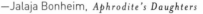

remain with (name of the mother-to-be) to give her all the courage she will need to birth her child. Spirit of the **East**, we thank you for your presence. You are free to leave our circle. Please remain with (name of the mother-to-be) so the burdens of mothering will become light as a feather."

ELEMENT-INSPIRED RELEASE: "This gathering is blessed with the gifts of the **North**. We give thanks for the firm foundation we find beneath us and the stable home to which we may return. Our lives are enriched by these gifts. We release you with our thanks. This gathering is blessed with the gifts of the **West**. We give thanks for the wonder and excitement we have shared today, for the refreshing cleansing we received by releasing what we no longer need, and for the deep commitments we have made. We release you with our thanks. This gathering is blessed with the gifts of the **South**. We give thanks for the warmth we feel for one another, which has created a new, sacred circle—a safe place for the heat of our heart's passion—and your light that does indeed brighten the darkest of times. We release you with our thanks. This gathering is blessed with the gifts of the **East**. We give thanks for the communication of the heart, mind, and body made possible here today and for our new knowledge of the

growth found in sharing silences. We have made fresh beginnings today as individuals and as a circle. We release you with our thanks."

CIRCLE-INSPIRED RELEASE: "We give thanks for the gifts of the **North**, for surrender, for death that allows change, and for the dark, quiet place of the womb time, where peace and wintry white purity allow for clarity. Thank you for making our sacred circle a firm foundation to stand upon today. We give thanks for the gifts of the **West**, whose all-encompassing sea indeed washed clean our circle and made way for our dreams and feelings to flow, so we in turn could grow. For this we are thankful. To the **South**, whose power is the sun, high in the sky, we give thanks. Your cleansing fire burned away what had no place here and made way for this circle's heart to become its hearth. Our passions are free to grow and glow bright and hot. We are grateful for your incredible blessings. And we are thankful for the bright and beautiful gifts of the **East**, whose driving winds carried away from our circle that which did not belong here. Your promise of first light with the rising of the sun helped open us. We give thanks that our circle is now a place for the wonderful communion of our hearts, our minds, and our souls."

WORKING WITH GOD, GODDESS, OR SPIRIT
God, Goddess, and Spirit are concepts of the Divine intended to connect us to a power greater than ourselves. The specific definitions of their attributes and expressions are of human creation and subject to interpretation. Whatever you call it and however you define it, the ineffable nature of divinity is available to us all. Intentionally making a connection with the Divine is a wonderful way to tap into the energies that are needed to give birth. By inviting a circle of women to make a connection with the Divine, the group energy is intensified and becomes an even greater gift to the mother-to-be.

When designing a blessingway ritual, appeal to the aspect of God, Goddess, or Spirit that will open the participants' hearts, minds, and bodies, thereby broadening the possibilities of support for the mother-to-be. The ways in which you can open yourselves to the Divine are as numerous as the peoples of the world and then some. By carefully selecting a form of Spirit that reaches the mother-to-be's heart—be it God, a specific goddess such as Demeter, or universal Spirit—you can help her make the best use of divine inspiration.

Creating Altars for God, Goddess, or Spirit
A central altar is built in honor of the form of the Divine you have chosen to

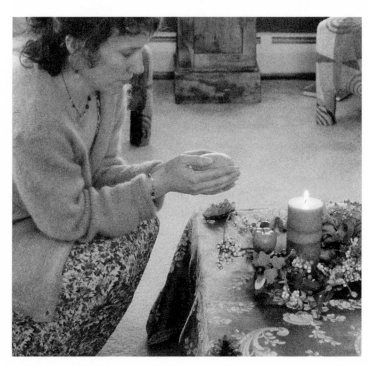

work with during your ritual. Located in the middle of the circle, it contains a variety of sacred symbols and provides a focal point for the women. A central altar should be present at every blessingway. It can be built on the floor or on a low table, depending upon your seating arrangement. What goes on this altar is entirely up to you. The central altar for one ritual may simply display a beautiful pillar candle (often gifted to the mother-to-be as an everlasting symbol of her connection to Spirit), while an altar at another ritual might also include the statue of a specific goddess, images of pregnant women, found objects symbolizing Mother Earth, and personal items that support each participant's work.

Your central altar should include an altar (or table) cloth, a vase of fresh flowers, and a new pillar candle (sometimes called a Spirit or Goddess candle). Beyond this, the nature of your ritual will determine the specific items to include.

A central altar usually includes images or symbols of the particular Divine energy that you will be summoning for the ritual. (See the appendix on page 117 to learn more.) If you will not be working with a specific deity, there are many alternative forms of the Divine to build altars for, including the following suggestions:

Mother Earth altar: This is a wonderful altar to create for women who feel a deep connection to nature. Mother Earth is often represented by the Greek goddess Gaia, so images and characteristics related to Gaia could be used. Try a nature-based altar covered with an abundance of fruits, flowers, nuts, seeds, and other treasures that come from the earth.

Mother within altar: This altar honors the inner wisdom of the mother-to-be (and all women). It speaks to the place deep within all of us that knows how to give birth to, how to care for, and how to guide our children. It is the place of our higher selves. Create this altar to symbolically support the idea that all we need to do is learn how to access the knowledge and wisdom we already carry within us. Request that guests loan or gift to the altar personal symbols that speak of inner wisdom, strength, and our nurturing

capacity as women.

Pregnancy and birth altar: This altar displays profound symbols and images of pregnancy, nursing, and motherhood, some of which are often present on the deity-inspired central altars of most blessingways. These special items symbolize the powers of strength, courage, and healing, upon which the mother-to-be will need to draw during her upcoming labor.

Mother or female ancestor altar: In honor of our female lineage, this beautiful altar hosts photos, cherished gifts, and items that symbolize the relationships we all have with our mothers, aunts, grandmothers, and great grandmothers.

Guests "in spirit" altar: This altar honors important people in the expectant mom's life who could not attend her blessingway. By placing a photograph of her special friend or family member (or an item that symbolizes them) on an altar, their presence can in essence be evoked.

Family or siblings altar: This altar includes photos of the mother-to-be's husband, partner, or other children, since they are generally not present at her blessingway. These photos can be a great focal point for her, especially if her family or the sibling(s)-to-be will be honored as part of her blessingway ritual.

Calling God, Goddess, or Spirit

Here are several examples for you to use, modify, or be inspired by as you set out to write your own invocation or evocation to the Divine. During the ritual, once you summon the presence of the Divine, light the pillar candle you have included on your central altar.

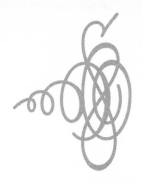
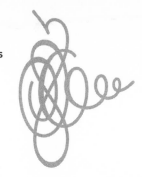

When the mother-to-be and participants are more comfortable with a traditional form of the Divine, you may call upon God to be present at the blessingway.

CALLING UPON GOD: "We open our hearts to the presence of God here today. O Holy One, may you guide our hearts and minds to the highest understanding of you, of love, so your loving inspiration may bless the purpose of our gathering. And may this gathering bring (name of the mother-to-be) a wealth of strength, peace, and joy to bless her way as she labors and mothers her children. Amen."

Many women choose to work with the feminine expression of the Divine known as the Goddess. One way to think about this form of divinity is as an archetype of the feminine spirit. We can summon her to join us in the general form of divine energy—the Goddess—or call upon one of her many specific faces—such as Demeter, Devi, or Kuan Yin—in recognition that she is the symbolic personification of qualities we have within ourselves. When we do this, these qualities become tangible and more easily accessed.

SUMMONING THE GODDESS: "We invite the Goddess to join us today. She is earth herself, her body reflecting mountains and valleys, fields and rivers. Her palpable sensuality is a celebration of physical existence. She represents the waves of primordial waters from which all life and consciousness arise. The great Goddess is woman's faceless, egoless, primal self. She is peaceful in her body and her truly miraculous power—as woman, as earth—to create life."

You may need to start by writing an informational summons (a simple fact-based introduction), if that's what you're most comfortable with. Here's an example:

SUMMONING DEMETER: "Demeter, the Greek goddess of grain, is said to be the most nourishing of all the mother goddesses. When the Romans adopted the myth of the gods, they renamed Demeter "Ceres," from whose name the word "cereal" is derived. Along with her nurturing characteristics, Demeter's true essence is the bond she holds with her daughter, Persephone. Demeter brings forth the fruits of the earth and facilitates the changing of the seasons. According to legend, when Demeter becomes separated from Persephone, the land becomes barren and we experience winter. But when reunited, spring arrives, and Demeter once again allows things to grow. Demeter, we request your presence. Please be with us today."

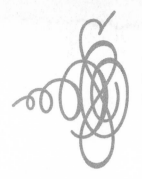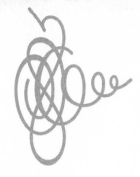

A SAFE CIRCLE HOLDS THE DREAM OF WHAT
[A WOMAN] COULD BE IN CONFIDENCE AND
NOURISHES THE POSSIBILITY.

—Jean Shinoda Bolen, *The Millionth Circle*

Or, you can move right into writing a more lyrical summons that sings the praises of the goddess whom you are calling. Here's an example:

SUMMONING DEMETER: "O Mother Demeter, come, gather us in your nurturing bosom; whisper to us soft joys of pregnancy. Bonded to you we are, your daughters. Nourish us, raise us, share with us your awe of this mother-to-be. O patient, caring Mother, come, return to us from shadowed lands beneath the reaches of the olive tree. Hear us now we are, your daughters. Leave your well of sorrow; remove your darkened cloak of grief. O Mother Demeter, come now; wake and tend your gardens for they have slept the winter long. Your sustenance we are, your daughters. Your everlasting love a gift, we wish to learn your song."

Great mothers are another feminine expression of Spirit you may call upon for your ritual. These mothers come to us in a wide variety of beautiful and powerful forms, and they journey to us from many different cultural traditions.

SUMMONING MOTHER EARTH: "Today we call upon the divine essence of Mother Earth. Within her, she holds all the wisdom of the world. Her harvest represents our abundance and fertility. Her very nature is the source of mothering and nurturing that we each carry within us. With the lighting of this candle, we invoke her spirit. Oh great Mother Earth, please be with us today."

ADDITIONAL WAYS OF OPENING TO THE DIVINE

Spirit presents itself in many different forms. There are other expressions of the Divine that may also be possibilities for the ritual you are designing. Archangels, saints, animals, ancestors, friends, family members, or the mother-to-be's older children may be incorporated into a blessingway in a way that reflects the mother-to-be's beliefs and desires in a personal and intimate way.

CHAPTER 5

Ritual Stage 2: Shifting

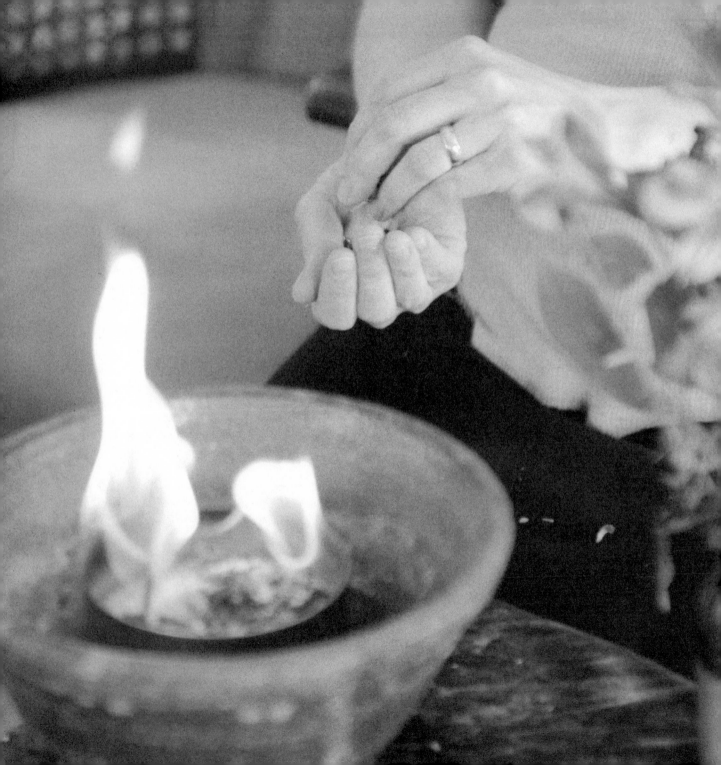

The Celtic **Spiral of Life** is a symbol of the oneness found in our connection with earth, with self, and with the Divine.

BY THIS POINT IN THE RITUAL, we will have created a sacred space, cleared away our cares, and formed our safe container. All the energies that we wish to have present to assist us with our ritual have been summoned, and the women in the circle are poised and ready to go. So now it's time to make the shift into the realm of circle consciousness.

We begin by becoming quiet and centered in ourselves. From there we become present to our purpose by stating our intentions for the gathering. After we have come into full awareness, we make a shift, tapping first into our collective feminine spirit and then into the mother-to-be's needs.

Stating the Purpose

State the purpose of your ritual to ensure that everyone, including Spirit, knows what you're trying to accomplish—what the mother-to-be would like help or support with. This is a great place to recap the ritual guidelines as well, especially if this is a first-time experience for any of the women in the circle. Each guest will play a vital role, so empower everyone by reaffirming the importance of their presence and the value of their contributions. Here's one version of a statement of purpose to help you compose your own:

We've gathered here today to acknowledge, honor, and celebrate Lillian's journey into motherhood. In this sacred space we've so lovingly created, we will help Lillian clear her path to motherhood by supporting her as she releases her fears, worries, and anything else that may stand in the way of her fully embracing the coming of her third child. By our coming together, we will also weave a web of support for Lillian, pledging our care and our willingness to provide for her throughout the weeks to come.

A blessingway is a sacred, Spirit-guided ritual. In light of this, we ask that everyone stay mindful, flexible, and speak consciously. We also ask that everyone stay present during the ritual, focusing your attention on Lillian and sending her your love and support while she is doing her work. We all have a lot going on in our lives, so if at any time you find that you become distracted by your own thoughts and feelings, please acknowledge them—but then put them away somewhere safe, so you can stay fully present for Lillian. You can use your breath to carry these thoughts and feelings away, or energetically send them down into the ground, into the arms of Mother Earth for safekeeping. The Grandmother Jar on the North altar is another safe place where you can energetically stow things away.

A blessingway has the power to evoke very deep emotions. Should Lillian (or anyone in the circle) become emotional, we ask that you not touch her nor offer her a tissue, unless she asks for it. Though well-intended, these offerings of comfort may actually shut down a wonderful release process. Lillian's blessingway is a no-fault ritual, so please do not be concerned if you've never been to a blessingway before. In this safe and sacred circle, all contributions will be honored. We do request that you maintain a thoughtful and reverent attitude, and that whatever you hear in this circle remains here. Confidentiality is key to creating safety for everyone today.

Our circle has been cast and is now closed. However, if you find you must leave the circle to take care of personal needs during our ritual, please feel free to do so. We just ask that you leave and return quietly. If anyone needs to leave the blessingway before it's over, we also ask that you leave quietly, observing ritual silence. Thank you for joining us.

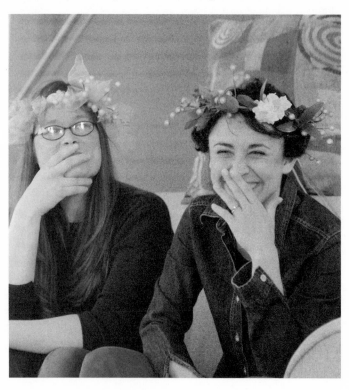

Introducing Participants

The circle has been cast, the guidelines repeated, and the purpose stated. Now it's time to unite the women who will be working together in the ritual. When blessingway participants come from different circles, include personal introductions as part of your format so no women are strangers to one another once the ritual begins. Personal introductions will really help unify a circle of women. There are many interesting (and fun!) ways to get to know one another.

Getting-to-know-you questions are quickly revealing. Have everyone tell about their favorite smells, childhood idols, or what they wanted to be when they grew up. Or, have each woman introduce herself by her matrilineal heritage: *"I am Barbara, daughter of*

Connecting

Connecting with one another in a circle is an element of transition. It is here that you move from simply being rooted in self to establishing your connection with one another and to your collective feminine spirit. It is also here that you get in sync with one another and with your common purpose.

Sharing food or drink is one way to connect. Eating from a common pot, pulling off a chunk of corn-bread, or sharing a cup of special tea—these are all wonderful ways to accomplish a shift in energy. Eating is very grounding, and it can be a helpful thing to do when transitions are being made. Indeed, many religious faiths share food to connect members to one another. Drinking a cup of tea together can also be an extremely mindful, meditative, and connective process.

Joanne, granddaughter of Lillian, great granddaughter of Lillian." If someone can't remember that far back, have them cite their female relations: *"I am Yana, mother of Claire and Lyra, sister of Marah, daughter of Kathleen, granddaughter of Claire and Julie."*

Without a doubt, it will be a powerful experience if each woman introduces herself by her connection with the mother-to-be: *"I am Shelly, and Jennifer and I have been friends since we were born—our mothers were best friends."* Or the women may share about the symbolic item they placed on the central altar: *"I am Tanya, and I brought the birth necklace that is made from the beads that were given to me at my blessingway. It gave me strength when I had my baby—because when I focused on it, I could really feel the support and presence of all the women who had contributed each bead."*

Meditation is another terrific way to form connections. You can incorporate a simple five-minute meditation or a more complex guided meditation that takes the circle of women on a journey that lasts for about thirty minutes. Here are several meditations that may work well during your ritual:

SILENT MEDITATION

Guide the circle of women to relax, get comfortable, and close their eyes. Then lead them to focus on the gentle rhythm of their breath. Next, invite them to open themselves up to the group and to feel themselves a part of it, letting the feelings and sensations of the experience flow through them. Pause for a while. Finally, when you are ready to end the meditation, guide them to slowly reopen their eyes and bring their awareness back to the room.

MUSIC MEDITATION

Invite the circle of women to relax, get comfortable, and close their eyes. As with silent meditation, lead the women to open themselves up to the sensations of the group and to feel themselves a part of it. Then guide them to listen closely to the sound of a heartbeat, a drum, a piece of beautiful music, or a song with meaningful and reflective words. Invite them to focus on the sound and to let it completely envelop them. As the music is ending, ask the women to slowly reopen their eyes and bring their awareness back to the room.

BIRTH STORY VISUALIZATION

You can ask the mother-to-be to write down her imagined birth story ahead of time, so you can read it aloud during the ritual. Guide the circle of women to relax, get comfortable, and close their eyes. Then ask them to visualize the story playing out (as you read it) to support and help manifest the mother-to-be's vision.

❀ . ❀ . ❀

There are many wonderful sources for meditations, but don't be afraid to create your own. The following

shell meditation is one that Barb crafted when she first started designing blessingways:

Sit or lie in a comfortable position, and bring your attention to your breath. Stay aware of your breath as it moves in and out of your body. With each exhalation, feel your body relax and your thoughts let go.

If thoughts or concerns do arise, surrender them and allow them to dissipate with your breath. Be aware of any physical tension in your body; breathe right into that spot, allowing your breath to massage and release any remaining tension. Keeping your focus on your breath and consciously remaining relaxed and open . . . bring all your attention within.

Now, imagine yourself on a beach—a beautiful, white-sand beach laden with shells. It is warm, and the water is softly lapping the sand, creating a soothing lullaby. You walk slowly down the beach in awe of Mother Earth's gifts, the beauty of the shells scattered all over the beach. Your eye fixes on one such treasure. You bend down and pick up an amazing shell and hold it in your hand. With reverence for its beauty, perfection, and grace, your eyes close, and you begin to dream. In this dream your shell begins to grow. It grows larger and larger until it is much larger than you. You circle the shell noticing with great awe the beauty reflected in its colors and textures—you are taken aback by its wholeness, as if it could in fact hold all the answers of the world.

As you walk further around the shell, you reach its entrance, which is now big enough for you to step into. The interior colors are vibrant, warm, and soft; the

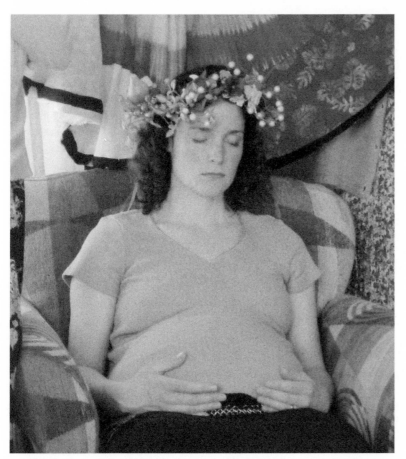

aware you are. Your breath is effortless, deep, and consistent, reminding you of the sound of the lapping waters outside the shell: a comforting, soothing lullaby connecting you to Spirit. As you spiral deeper and deeper inside the shell, you feel more and more relaxed. Worries and fears drop away with each step.

Now (name of the mother-to-be), become aware that the comfort, safety, and love—the sense of connection you are experiencing—must be just how your baby feels being cradled in your womb. Warm, nourished, nurtured. The sound of a mother's heartbeat and breath are all that is, and all that is needed.

After spiraling deeper and deeper, you reach the innermost chamber, the very center of the shell. It feels so comfortable and safe here that you curl up into a fetal position, cradled by the walls of this soft center. The only audible sound is your breath as it washes in and out.

texture as smooth as silk. As you enter the shell, you immediately feel warm and safe. Reverence overcomes you as you realize you are entering a sacred sanctuary.

You walk with great awareness deep into the shell— aware of each footstep you take on the shell's smooth interior. The deeper you walk, the more present and

Now (name of the mother-to-be), imagine the shell filling with all your closest friends, loved ones, ancestors, angels, and spirit guides. They are spiraling, circling, and surrounding you, —offering protection and sending love and blessings. For those of you who have journeyed here with (name of the mother-to-be),

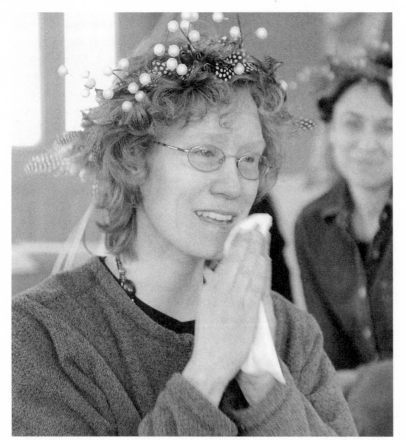

Place one hand over your heart and your other hand over your baby's heart. Notice the exchange of energy between you. Be aware that this pulsating energy is love, and as it fills your body and travels down your arms and into your hands, allow it to flow freely between your body and your baby.

Your baby is smiling with reassurance, knowing what a wonderful and loving mother you are. Take a moment to say what is in your heart, to ask any questions you may have for your baby. (Pause.) Now listen to what your baby has to communicate to you. (Pause.) Your baby feels so safe, secure, and loved in your womb. And you too feel safe, secure, and loved in the womb of support created by your friends, loved ones, and guides. Take a deep breath, and breathe this in. Fully absorb how much you are loved and supported.

For your infant, knowing this love and security makes entering this world safe and desirable. And for you (name of the mother-to-be), feeling this love, confidence, and support leaves you empowered with the qualities and strength needed to give birth—gently, lovingly, and successfully.

You recognize it is time to journey back. (Name of mother-to-be), say good-bye to your baby and reas-

consciously visualize the safe container you are forming for her. Send her your love and blessings.

(Name of the mother-to-be), feeling so deeply connected to all that is and all those in your life who love and support you, begin to see how connected your baby is to you. Allow yourself to truly take in how deeply bonded you already are. Tap into this magical place.

sure him or her of your connection. Tell your baby, "I can't wait to hold you in my arms." Thank your circle of support and follow them as they tunnel out of the shell, slowly returning to this world. Let us all carry these feelings of great love and connection with us, all the way back to this very room. Before we open our eyes, let's take in a deep breath to anchor our feelings of love and connection. Slowly breathe out. (Name of the mother-to-be), know that whenever you feel the need for support, it is as close as your breath—breathing in, and breathing out. Now let us all begin to turn our attention gently to our bodies. When you feel fully present to yourself, here in this room, slowly open your eyes, allowing them to gradually adjust to the light.

Releasing Fears

During this segment of the shifting stage, you fully commit yourselves to being present to your purpose by releasing fears (or anything else that might distract you, cloud your efforts, or block your intentions). The process of letting go of fear is usually one of the most powerful parts of a blessingway ritual—for both the mother-to-be and the women who have come to support her.

Expressing fears helps participants let them go, releasing them from the

Make Your Own Fear-Releasing Herb Mix
Many common herbs carry properties you'll want to include in your herbal releasing mixture. Lavender, fennel, chamomile, rose petals, clove, parsley, sage, rosemary, and thyme are thought to carry cleansing, protective, healing, wishful, and loving energies. Mix herbs in any proportion or combination to produce a fragrant and symbolically powerful mixture.

women's hearts and placing them in the hands of Spirit. Expressing fear is not the same as giving energy to it; in fact, it is the opposite. For when you deny that your fear exists, you leave it locked up deep within yourself—in a dark, cool, damp place—giving it the perfect conditions in which to grow. Having the women release their fears and expectations creates space within them—space that can then be filled with wishes, blessings, and other positive love-centered energies through the remaining work of the blessingway.

Because of the fear-releasing segment's power (and for the great benefit of all the women who are present), blessingway participants should be encouraged to release their fears aloud, though you may also invite guests to release silently if that is more comfortable for them. It is helpful to ask a participant who has already experienced releasing her fear in a ritual to go first, as she can help alleviate uncertainty by acting as a model for the rest of the women to follow. Two types of fear-releasing rituals follow.

THE BURNING RITUAL
A burning ritual is a dramatic and effective way to release fear, and it can actually be done indoors if you

have a fireplace or create a smokeless flame. Along with a fire, you'll also need to have on hand a bowl of special fear-releasing herbs (see sidebar for recipe) to pass around the circle. Once the fire is going, beginning with the mother-to-be, invite each woman to: take a pinch of herbs from the bowl in turn; approach the fire; state the fear, expectation, or distraction that she wishes to let go of; drop the herbs into the flame; and return to her seat in the circle. You can go around the circle as many times as you've allotted time for.

To use the smokeless flame method, place a clean tuna can in a fireproof bowl. Set the bowl on a trivet (or something similar) to protect the surface it's sitting on. Fill the tuna can half to three-fourths full with Epsom salts. Pour in rubbing alcohol just to cover the salts. Light the mixture carefully. (You'll want to set this up on a sturdy board or table somewhere near the center of your circle.) When the fire is going, starting with the mother-to-be, have the women release their fears along with the herbs into the fire. You may need to relight the fire several times, depending upon how long the fear-releasing segment takes, since the alcohol will burn off, and the herbs may build up and eventually smother the flames. When you are sure the flame is completely out, carefully pour a little more alcohol over the salt and herbs in the tuna can, and relight carefully.

For an outdoor burning ritual, arrange to have someone go out to start your fire ahead of time, so it's ready when the circle regroups around the fire pit (or fireproof bowl). Release any of the following items into the flames to symbolize the women's fears, ex-pectations, or distractions: bits of wood, small sticks, branches, wood shims, pine cones, sprays of dried herbs, a pinch of fear-releasing herbal mixture, slips of paper containing written fears, or small (nontoxic!) symbolic objects that will burn easily. End with the following closing statement: *"By burning these things, we release our fears, expectations, and distractions to the four winds. May we now be free to focus our minds and hearts upon the present moment."*

THE WORRY JAR RITUAL

Also called the God Jar, Goddess Jar, or Grandmother Jar, the Worry Jar can be any kind of container. The only requirement is that it should have a lid, so it may effectively contain all the fears, expectations, distractions, and worries that are released into it. This releasing activity is not as dramatic as a burning ritual, but it is very effective nevertheless. Give each woman in the circle several slips of paper and a pen to write down her fears and worries. Pass the jar around the circle, and invite each woman to read (in turn) one of her fears aloud, then fold the paper and place it in the worry jar for safekeeping. Continue going around the circle until all fears have been placed in the jar. Using this fear-releasing technique tends to take more time than a burning ritual, so keep this in mind when designing your ritual.

The bits of paper in the Worry Jar should be disposed of after the blessingway is over (unless you plan to revisit them at a later date). This can be done effectively by burying the paper slips in the ground or by burning them and then burying or scattering the ashes.

CHAPTER 6

Ritual Stage 3: Focusing

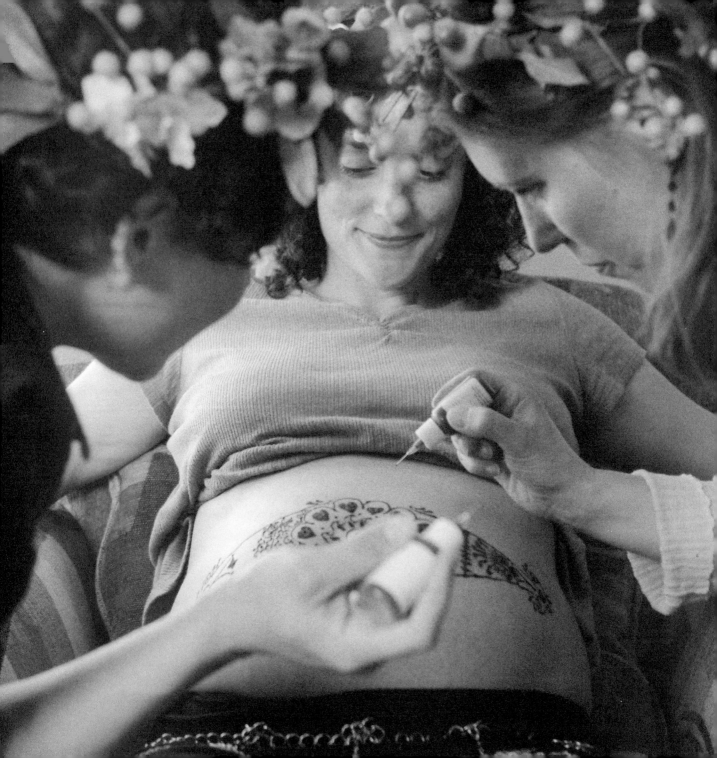

Hecate's Wheel is an ancient Greek symbol that represents
the three phases of the moon (waxing, waning, full) and of womankind
(maiden, mother, crone).

FOCUSING IS THE STAGE where we do the work specific to our gathering. Here our attention turns to honoring, pampering, and preparing the mother-to-be for her journey into motherhood. The ritual elements and activities we choose to include reflect the mother-to-be's desires and address any concerns she may have about birth or becoming a mother.

To give birth, a woman must let go. Perhaps for the first time in her life, she will learn the lesson of what it truly means to surrender to something greater than herself. The birth process, like breathing, happens on its own. A mother-to-be must be willing to openly trust and surrender so the birth can unfold from deep within her.

The blessingway ritual as a whole (and in particular, honoring and pampering the mother-to-be) can introduce the mother-to-be to deep surrender, such as she will experience when giving birth. Receiving intimate attention is a wonderful exercise in trust. Women who are being pampered sometimes start out feeling self-conscious or tense, as many of us are not used to being the star of the show. Being honored, even doted on, by a room full of women can feel uncomfortable and awkward. However, such compassionate pampering as a gentle massage or the warm water of a footbath will help the mother-to-be

to relax. As she slowly surrenders to the circle's loving hands, she'll begin to let go, entrusting herself to the women who envelop her—and beyond, to the open arms of divine grace.

Honoring

For the honoring segment of the blessingway, seat the mother-to-be in a place of prominence set within the circle. Most of the honoring activities will have been prepared in advance (having been announced on the invitation). Introduce the honoring activities now, and invite the guests to present their warm wishes and bright blessings. The mother-to-be can be honored in a variety of ways; several suggestions follow.

BELLY CASTING

An amazing—though messy—experience, belly casting is a fun way to honor and preserve a pregnant silhouette. You can choose to either create a belly cast or decorate a belly cast during the ritual. (A cast needs to dry for one week before it is ready to adorn.) Buy a kit or collect the materials yourself. (See the Casting a Belly sidebar for supplies you will need and for casting instructions.)

Casting a Belly

Casting a mother-to-be's belly will require approximately one hour of uninterrupted time. You will need one or more people to help with the casting.

First, locate the following materials:

- A chair, if the mother-to-be opts for a seated position
- One to two large pieces of plastic (or tarps) to use as drop cloths
- Scissors
- Six to eight rolls of fast-drying plaster bandages (available at craft or medical supply stores)
- A shallow pan (a 9 by 13-inch baking pan works well)
- Enough petroleum jelly (or earth-friendly alternative) to coat the entire area to be cast
- A roll of paper towels to wipe hands or spills

Next, prepare yourself, your space, and your supplies:

- Dress in old clothes, so if the plaster drips, it will not matter. Short-sleeved shirts are also a must, as long sleeves tend to get in the way. Remove all jewelry and watches.
- Spread out drop cloths over the entire area where you will be working, including the chair (if choosing a seated position).
- Cut plaster bandages into 6- to 8-inch-long strips.
- Fill pan with warm water.

Then, prepare the mother-to-be:

- Her belly and torso should be bare, and she should wear old clothes on the rest of her body or none at all. She should also remove all jewelry and watches.
- Have her experiment with poses, striking several like a model. Take your time selecting a pose that she not only likes, but will be comfortable holding for at least thirty minutes. (She could stand, sit, lean forward, lean back, twist slightly, wrap her arms under her belly, and so on.) Provide her with a mirror so she can examine her pose, posture, and position. This representation of her pregnant silhouette will last a long time, so help her choose a pose that will fully portray her beautiful goddess body.
- Use petroleum jelly to liberally coat her belly, breasts, sides of torso, and any other body parts that will be cast.

Now, create the belly cast:

- Using a process that is similar to creating papier-mache, dip the plaster strips into the warm water one at a time, taking care not to let any strip fold or twist. Run the strip through two fingers, wringing out the excess water. If a strip does fold, twist, or wrinkle, be sure to straighten it out before applying it to the belly.
- Place strips all over the desired area, overlapping and carefully smoothing out each one. Be sure to tuck the strips in close around the mother-to-be's breasts and take care not to leave any gaps. Cover her entire torso area, but only halfway around her sides. (If you place the strips too far around toward

her back, you will not be able to get her out of the cast!) Work quickly, yet carefully, as the plaster will begin to dry in about fifteen minutes and then start pulling away from her body. Apply three to five layers of the plaster strips.

- Once you have achieved the desired thickness, let the plaster dry for about fifteen minutes. As it dries, the cast will start to pull away from the mother-to-be's skin on its own.

- Remove the cast carefully. Help the mother-to-be wiggle out while you support the cast. Be mindful that some of her pubic and/or underarm hairs may have adhered to the plaster and may pull (and hurt) when the cast is removed.

Let the cast dry completely (for a full week). Then decorate the belly cast:

- Once it's dry, smooth the cast's surface by sanding it lightly. If you prefer, you may coat it with a layer of plaster of paris (you'll need to let the plaster dry for a few more days in this case).

- Prime the cast with a coat of gesso, if desired.

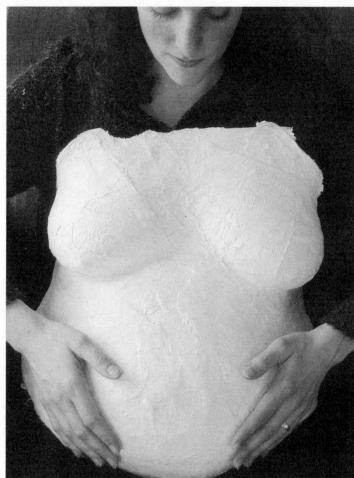

- Adorn the cast with paint, découpage, beads, stones, and so on.

- Seal the cast with shellac.

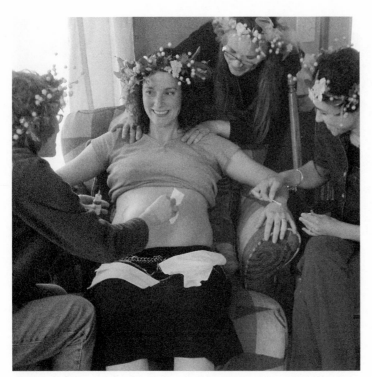

the child all about his or her very special mother. This is a very deep, meaningful, and moving way to honor the mother-to-be, and reading their letters can be a way to include friends or family members who could not attend the ritual.

INSPIRATIONAL STORYTELLING

Guests are invited to share a personal story or a reading that speaks to the mother-to-be's personal journey. Poems, prose, quotes, affirmations, songs, prayers, and biblical passages are all great sources from which to draw.

❀ . ❀ . ❀

Oftentimes, the mother-to-be wishes to do some honoring herself! She may want to speak from her heart or read from her journal about her own mother, grandmother, friends, or children. Small

CROWNING

A crown or headpiece is a mark of distinction, showing that the bearer holds divine attributes. A pregnant woman is a sacred vessel, and crowning her heightens her awareness of this. Crowns or headpieces can be as simple as floral wreaths or as elaborate as jeweled tiaras.

LETTERS TO THE BABY

Composed ahead of time by each guest, these letters are addressed to the baby-to-be. Read aloud, they tell

ceremonies, such as the sibling ceremony, can be created to provide her the special time she needs. During the sibling ceremony, we have witnessed women speak beautifully from their hearts, read from their previous pregnancy journals, and share letters they have written directly to their existing children. This ceremony is often a very powerful experience for everyone in the circle. Invite the mother-to-be to bring a photo of her child(ren) to the blessingway ritual, so she may "hold them" while she is speaking.

Pampering

Pampering is one of the most important elements of a blessingway. It not only physically prepares the mother-to-be, it also enables participants to communicate their support and care to her in ways that words cannot. The activities you engage in carry deep symbolic meaning and help the mother-to-be feel relaxed as well.

Every woman in the circle needs to place her loving hands tenderly on the mom-to-be in some way. It's often impossible for everyone to pamper the mother-to-be at one time; therefore, the guests may need to rotate to different modes every five to ten minutes. While some women are physically brushing the mother-to-be's hair, massaging her shoulders, bathing her feet, rubbing lotions into her skin, applying henna, or sending blessings, others may share personal stories, insights, or selected readings from their place in the circle. You can also "nourish" the mom-to-be by providing her with food and drink, or even feeding her if her hands are otherwise engaged. Regardless of the specific task each guest is engaged in, every woman in the circle should remain focused on the mother-to-be. Along with the other pampering elements you select for the mother-to-be, feel free to incorporate each of these symbolic activities into your ritual.

Herbal Footbath Recipe
Any combination of the following herbs and flowers (dried or fresh) will produce a fragrant, soothing, and symbolically potent footbath: chamomile, lavender, fennel seeds, lemon verbena, rose petals or buds, sage, coriander, borage, rosemary, or red raspberry leaf.

HAIR BRUSHING

Brushing the mother-to-be's hair untangles any snarls, symbolically straightening out anything left undone in order to ensure a smooth labor. It is also said that changing one's hairdo denotes a woman's passage from maidenhood to motherhood. Loose hair may be braided or put up in a more mature style to symbolize this passage. Or, let her hair down to symbolize letting go.

MASSAGE

Massaging the mother-to be's shoulders prepares her for bearing the responsibility of motherhood. Massaging her hands readies her for the physically hard work of motherhood. Massaging her feet enables her to continue on her journey. Use a softly scented lotion or massage oil, gently working it into her arms as well as her hands.

FOOT BATHING

A footbath honors a woman's "own two feet"—on which she will have to stand in order to care for another human being. Some believe a foot bathing washes away girlhood, making way for motherhood. It definitely soothes the mother-to-be's feet, clearing the way for a peaceful journey. Place a tub of comfortably warm water and herbs (see the Herbal Footbath Recipe sidebar) at her feet, then let her feet soak while she's receiving massages and having her hair brushed. Provide a bar of natural soap, so her feet may be washed as well, and use lotion to moisturize them after they've been dried.

Adorning

Adorning is one of our favorite ritual elements! It can really make the mother-to-be feel special, and it also lends itself to having all the women in the circle participate. Of all the methods listed below, mehndi is the one that we incorporate most often into our blessingway rituals. Plan to include at least one of the following activities in your blessingway.

CREATING MEHNDI ART

Mehndi is the ancient art of henna body painting. Not only are the results beautiful, but the process is creative and fun. Mehndi is traditionally practiced in India, Africa, and the Middle East, where the henna plant is believed to bring love, luck, protection, and good fortune. It is used for weddings, important rites of passage, and times of joyous celebration. Applying henna can be especially meaningful if each woman present takes a turn adding something to the mother-to-be's mehndi design. You can find mehndi kits at many natural food stores. (See page 141 for more information and additional sources.)

APPLYING BINDIS

Bindis are small, self-adhesive jewels that adhere easily to the skin. They are traditionally (but not exclu-sively) placed in the middle of the forehead. Originally based on a Hindu religious practice, bindis mark the spot between the eyebrows that is believed to be our gateway to the Divine (sometimes called our third eye). Available at most East Indian grocery stores or gift shops, they are a fun, inexpensive, and easy-to-use form of adornment.

PRESENTING CLOTHING

You can dress the mother-to-be in a special item of clothing that symbolically marks her transition from maiden to mother or that outfits her for her journey. A shawl, cape, or other beautiful piece of clothing can work wonderfully. We know someone who makes custom birthing gowns for women to wear during labor. Presenting the mother-to-be with such a gown at her blessingway may be especially touching.

BRAIDING AND BEADING HAIR

If the mother-to-be has long hair, tiny braids can be woven into it and then secured at the end with colorful beads. Infuse the beads with affirmations and blessings to deepen the experience. Weaving ribbons or dried flowers into her hair will look and feel lovely as well.

Giving Gifts

When you come together for a blessingway, it is a time to celebrate your diversity and to honor the distinctly different gifts and talents you each bring with you. Reflective of this, the gifts you offer to the mother-to-be during her blessingway will often hold little monetary value, but are heart-centered and rich in meaning.

Gift giving often flows nicely right after pampering and adorning. The only downside to this is that it will take place during a time when the mother-to-be is in an ultra-relaxed, almost euphoric state. Which, of course, is wonderful (and exactly where you want her to be!), but it does result in her memory of this part of her ritual being more dreamlike. Bearing this in mind, assign someone to act as a scribe and take on the very important task of writing down each gift that the mother-to-be receives, who it came from, and what meaning it holds.

Blessingway gifts are usually symbolic in nature, so guide guests ahead of time to choose an item or items that support the mother-to-be's needs. Everyone in the circle will enjoy watching and listening to each woman as she presents her gift and shares its significance with the mother-to-be. You will be consistently amazed by how creative and thoughtful these gifts are. Be sure to allot ample time for the gift-giving segment, as it tends to take quite a while to get around the circle.

Receiving so many gifts that have come from each guest's heart and soul may be an overwhelming experience for the mother-to-be. To help ensure that she stays present to the experience, minimize potential distractions by inviting the circle of guests to keep

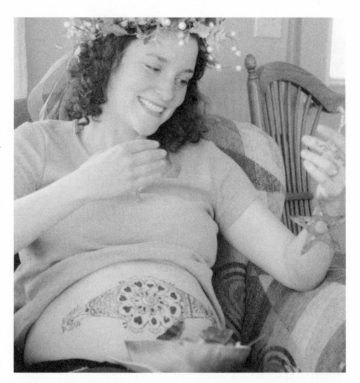

their full attention on the woman presenting her gifts, refraining from holding any side conversations or leaving the circle.

Symbolic gifts are very personal by design. They are given to bless, inspire, encourage, empower, acknowledge, welcome, bestow wishes, reaffirm connections, or honor the recipient's journey. They might come in the form of beads, cards, letters, poems, songs, jewelry, personal items from past or present, or even a once-coveted toy of a guest's own child. Found objects, childhood trinkets, cherished treasures, things

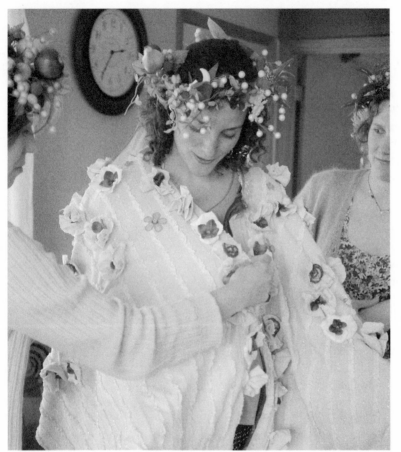

pleted at a later date. Collective gift making can be easily incorporated into the ritual as a group activity. One way to do this is by having each participant present their component to the mother-to-be and then add it to the collective creation while the next participant is presenting her gift. This keeps the mother-to-be engaged in the activity without becoming involved in the actual gift-making process. The completed group gift can be presented at the end of the ritual segment, or after the ritual, should a finishing touch be required.

In addition to symbolic and collective gifts, guests frequently offer a postpartum gift of service to the new mother. The choice of a postpartum gift is generally left up to each individual, though very often the mother-to-be will request prepared meals. Looking for more ideas? Consider these postpartum

from nature, and even well-loved hand-me-downs make wonderful blessingway gifts.

You may also consider asking blessingway participants to contribute a component for a larger, group gift. This collective gift can be created prior to the blessingway, constructed as part of the ritual, or com-

offers: delivering prepared meals, running errands, shopping for groceries, cleaning the house, doing laundry, caring for pets, helping with projects, providing massages, photographing certain events, planning outings or activities for older children, providing breastfeeding support, spending time holding the baby

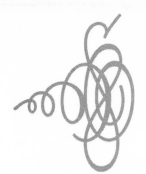
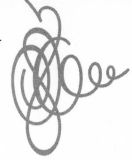

MOTHERING IS A SUBTLE ART WHOSE RHYTHM WE COLLECT
AS MUCH FROM ONE ANOTHER AS BY INSTINCT.
—Louise Erdrich, *The Blue Jay's Dance: A Birth Year*

(so the new mom may take a nap or a shower), or helping with birth announcements.

GIFTS FOR THE MOTHER-TO-BE

Gift-giving presents you with a terrific opportunity to tap into and express your creative selves. Not everyone feels artistic, but when participants allow themselves to create—and their creations come from their heart—all the women become artists, poets, and musicians. Whether the gift is an individual creation or a collective gift, knowing that all the participants poured their hearts and souls into the process will make it enduringly special for the mother-to-be. The end result doesn't have to be aesthetically correct to be beautiful and amazing in her eyes. Several gift ideas intended to keep your creative juices flowing follow.

Affirmations Poster

When we give birth, we're supposed to get out of our heads and get in touch with our bodies. Perhaps that's why it's so hard to remember to breathe! Affirmation posters are loving, supportive, and powerful ticklers that the mother-to-be can have with her when she gives birth. These posters incorporate words and images that can help her recall those important birthing concepts—squat…breathe…tone…open—during

labor. Bring an assortment of art supplies to the blessingway, such as: poster board, paints, pastels, pens, glitter, and collage materials to the ritual, then invite participants to get creative.

Altar in a Box

An altar in a box is a gift with spirit for a mother-to-be who is planning a hospital or birthing center delivery. The box itself might hold some significance, or it can be made meaningful when collectively adorned by the guests. Choose a fairly small container (no larger than a shoebox), so it can be packed in her overnight bag. Include a candle, a small cloth, affirmation cards, and small symbolic items or trinkets.

Birth Pouch

A birth pouch is a potent talisman for the mom-to-be. The bag can be purchased or made by hand and filled with small trinkets and items that represent characteristics, values, wishes, blessings—just about anything that will help the mother-to-be with the task that lies ahead of her.

Blessing Basket

Adorn a basket and fill it with eggs decorated with affirmations, blessings, quotes, personal messages, and

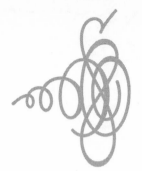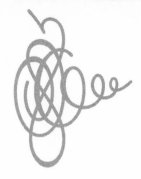

OUR DESIRE FOR PROTECTION, REASSURANCE, AND BLESSING
IS STRONG THROUGHOUT PREGNANCY AND BIRTH.

—Starhawk, Diane Baker, and Anne Hill, *Circle Round*

birth images. Be sure to blow out the eggs so they don't spoil. Or simply use cheery plastic Easter eggs, place inspirational quotes and affirmations inside them, and set them in your basket. (We hid an entire basket of plastic eggs around the house of one mom-to-be who was planning a home birth, so she could go on an inspirational Easter egg hunt while in labor!)

Blessingway Jewelry

Unique beads and semiprecious stones combine to make stunning bracelets, anklets, or necklaces. Craft pieces of love-filled jewelry for mothers-to-be, babies-to-be, and siblings-to-be. A wisdom necklace is a simple variation on this theme. Invite each guest to provide a bead that represents an important event that occurred during the mother phase (or other important phase if she's not a mother) of her life, and the wisdom she acquired as a result. Have each guest share their bead's significance as they string it onto a piece of jewelry wire, so their wisdom can be passed on to the mother-to-be in the form of a beautiful necklace.

Blessingway Scrapbook

Present the mother-to-be with a thoughtfully embellished scrapbook in which she can safely keep her cards, letters, written blessings, and small gifts. The guests can contribute decorative items and help embellish the scrapbook itself, or they can provide the special items it will contain.

Gifts from Nature

A tree, plant, or garden nursery gift certificate is a terrific gift for a mother-to-be who intends to eventually plant her baby's placenta in her yard. Trees have deep-rooted symbolic meaning, so it can be fascinating to research the qualities associated with each distinct variety.

Wreath or Headpiece

A beautiful wreath or headpiece is a wonderful blessingway keepsake. Made from fresh or dried flowers contributed by each guest, this ring of flora can be assembled during the blessingway, or it can be constructed ahead of time and presented to the mom-to-be as a crown during her ceremony.

GIFTS FOR FAMILY MEMBERS

There are times when it is important to recognize the baby-to-be, siblings-to-be, or family-to-be with a special gift during the blessingway. Several interesting ideas follow.

Baby Quilt

This is quite a gift! It does, however, require that someone with quilting skills take charge of managing the project and constucting the quilt. Choose a theme for the quilt, then request that each guest contribute a fourth of a yard of new or used fabric. Fabric squares should carry some significance, due to their design or origin. The quilt should be planned out and assembled ahead of time and then presented at the blessingway. You may also want to consider making a scrapbook to accompany the quilt. This scrapbook becomes the quilt's legend, containing a piece of each fabric along with a written explanation of who the fabric came from and what it symbolizes. (If desired, ask participants to supply enough fabric to enable you to do this.)

Family Unity Pouches

No one wants to feel like an outsider. When the mother-to-be is concerned that some family members will feel overshadowed by the new baby, try making potent little medicine bags for each family member. Fill the pouches with an array of small of items that symbolize values and ideals central to the family unit (for example, communication, trust, growth, or nurturing). Include in each bag one piece of a symbolic item that has been broken into as many parts as there are family members. This object is of particular

significance since it can be made complete only when all family members are together.

Mobile

Babies are mesmerized by mobiles. String together small symbolic trinkets, objects from nature, or just about anything that is colorful and attention grabbing to make a meaningful gift for the baby.

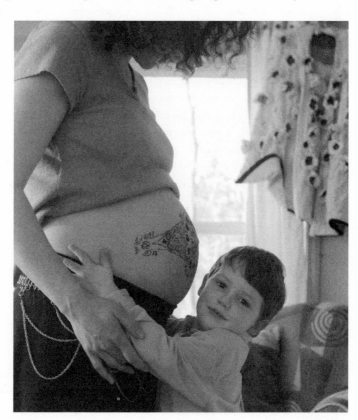

Making Jewelry

It's not too difficult to put together a piece of jewelry, but it does require a bit of creativity and planning, plus some specific supplies.

You will need the following:

- The mother-to-be's gift beads
- Filler beads (optional)
- Jewelry wire
- Scissors
- Two crimp beads
- One clasp
- Needle-nose pliers (for squeezing the crimp beads)
- One split ring (do not use a jump ring, as jump rings can pull open too easily)

Follow these steps to create a bracelet, anklet, or necklace:

1. Determine the size. Measure the mom-to-be's wrist or use a bracelet she already owns (or necklace or anklet) as a guide to determine the right length for your piece of jewelry.

2. Lay out her gift beads. On a piece of white cloth, line up the beads that the mom-to-be received as gifts. Arrange the beads in a pleasing way (graduated, by color, and so on).

3. Choose filler beads. We usually use small glass beads or seed beads as filler beads between the gift beads in order to set them off from one another. If you have a large number of gift beads and setting them apart is not possible, make a necklace instead of a bracelet or anklet or make two separate bracelets or anklets. The length of the piece of jewelry you are creating and the number and size of gift beads will dictate how many filler beads you need to space out the gift beads. Once you are happy with the layout, spacing, and design of your piece of jewelry, you are ready to string the beads.

4. String the beads. To string your piece of jewelry, measure out the desired length of jewelry wire, plus an extra three to four inches. (Having this extra wire to work with will make it much easier to add your clasp later on.) Cut the length you want with your scissors. Thread a small bead on the line and bring it to the end of your wire. Tie a knot around that small bead so it cannot fall off the wire. (This will temporarily prevent any beads from coming off the wire.) String your beads onto the wire in the order that you laid them out. Once they are all on the wire, check the length and the design, and make any necessary adjustments. Even with careful planning, the jewelry we make isn't always quite right the first time. We've found it's easiest to make adjustments (especially to the length of the piece) when we snip off the knotted bead and then add or remove beads from either end.

5. Add a crimp bead and a clasp. Thread a crimp bead on the end of the wire, then add your clasp. Now bring the wire back through the crimp bead and pull about one and a half inches of wire through the bead. Pull the crimp bead close to the clasp and pinch it with your needle-nose pliers. This will secure the clasp. Thread the end of the wire back through at least one-half inch of beads, then trim off the extra wire with your scissors. (Be sure to leave enough wire to easily add the split ring at the other end.)

6. Add another crimp bead and a split ring. On the other end, cut your original knot off if you haven't already, then thread on a crimp bead and a split ring. Thread the end of the wire back through the crimp bead and about one-half inch of the beads. Pull the end of the wire so you take up any remaining slack. (This is the most difficult part. You don't want to see extra wire and have beads floating around, nor do you want to pull it so tight that the bracelet or necklace buckles.) Once you feel that you have adequately taken up the slack, pinch the crimp bead with your needle-nose pliers. Trim off the extra wire with your scissors.

Nursing Box

Put together a very special nursing box for a toddler sibling. Full of toys, books, and interesting items, this nifty box can be set out when mom is nursing the new baby. This is a fascinating distraction, and toddlers will feel better when they too have something nurturing and fun to focus their attention on.

Super Big Brother or Super Big Sister Cape

Every child wants to be a superhero, especially in the eyes of his or her younger siblings. Why not whip up a playful yet powerful cape embellished with pieces of fabric, trim, patches, jewels, rhinestones . . . whatever! This gift honors the sibling in his or her new role as big brother or big sister.

Sharing and Storytelling

Wisdom comes in many forms and sometimes from unlikely places. It is often a very powerful experience for everyone in the circle when you share your stories with one another. Each participant has a tale or two to tell: tales of strength, love, and courage; tales of birth, bonding, and parenting. You can tell about yourselves, your families, or your great grandmother who birthed sixteen children. The stories you share should in some way honor the inherent power of women, leading the circle to a place of surrender, trust, and triumph.

A circle of women can spend hours sharing and telling their stories—it can be a ritual in itself! Incorporate sharing and storytelling into your blessing-

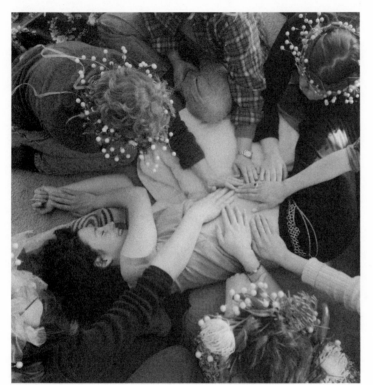

please) and set time parameters so the topics remain inspirational and no one feels cut off. It may also be wise to start the sharing process with someone who is familiar with circle work, as she can set the appropriate tone for the others to follow.

Blessings and Wishes

During a blessingway, there are many opportunities to offer blessings to the mother-to-be and her baby. Your individual blessings are often embedded in the gifts you bring or the activities in which you participate. Blessings may also be given in creative and powerful ways as a group. The following are some of the many touching ways in which you can lovingly bless the mother-to-be.

BLESSING PLEDGE

"Pledge to My Children" from the book *Celebrating Motherhood* by Andrea Alban Gosline, Lisa Burnett Bossi, and Ame Mahler Beanland, is a thoughtful, powerful, and beautiful blessing. When adapted slightly, it can be read aloud to the mother-to-be in unison. (See the Pledge to My Children sidebar.)

BLESSINGS BOX OR BASKET

Similar to a blessingway scrapbook, a blessings box or basket is specially created to hold inspirational quotes, affirmations, wishes, tokens, symbolic items, cards,

way as a defined segment, weave it in during pampering and adorning, or use it as a tool to help you keep the ritual flowing during any waiting periods (for instance, when the mom-to-be leaves the circle to visit the rest room).

A mother-to-be is often bombarded with tales of horror throughout her pregnancy, so make a concerted effort not to bring them into your sacred space. When inviting women to share, it's best to offer some guidelines (such as, positive experiences only,

Pledge to My Children

May you anticipate your child's birth, her childhood, and her life and encourage her to look forward too.

May you watch her flourish and discover her home in this magnificent world.

May you nurture her innocence and never forget the sacred place it comes from.

May you show her the way of wonder and walk along beside her.

May you stand for her as a parent and a friend, valuing her dreams just as you value your own.

May you voice your feelings honestly, and honor the promises you make.

May you listen to her thoughtfully and give her the freedom to expand her own mind.

May you envision her happy future, always mindful of the precious, present moment.

May you embrace her and enjoy her with your heart open wide.

—Andrea Alban Gosline, Lisa Burnett Bossi,
   and Ame Mahler Beanland, *Celebrating Motherhood*

candle (or Goddess candle), and place it on the central altar. (This is usually done near the end of the ritual, so the candles don't burn down too far.) At the end of the ritual, the candles are snuffed. The candles may remain with the mother-to-be, or the guests may take the candle they brought with them back home again. In either case, they are lit again when the mother-to-be goes into labor, as a symbol of the circle's support.

LAYING-ON-OF-HANDS BLESSING

Invite the women of the circle to gather around the mother-to-be and lovingly place their hands on her. They may take turns offering verbal blessings to her (as well as to the baby that lies sleeping in her womb), while maintaining physical contact for the duration of this activity.

and blessings for the mother-to-be and her baby. Go around the circle, inviting guests to offer their blessings and then place their special items in the blessings container.

CANDLE BLESSING

Ask guests to bring a votive candle to the ritual. Have each woman offer her wish or blessing to the mother-to-be, light her votive from the central pillar

ROSE WATER OR SALT WATER BLESSING

Salt water is often used for blessings because of its purifying qualities. Rose water is chosen at times to symbolize love, friendship, luck, and protection. There is a popular pagan self-blessing that works well if you choose a water blessing. Read the blessing aloud, and dip your fingers into the salt water or rose water before you touch each named part of the mother-to-be's body. (See the Pagan Self-Blessing sidebar.)

Pagan Self-Blessing

Divine Mother,

Bless (name of the mother-to-be), for she is your child.

(Dip fingers, touch crown.)

Bless (name of the mother-to-be)'s sight

that she may clearly see your path as well as her own.

(Dip fingers, touch forehead.)

Bless (name of the mother-to-be)'s throat

that she may speak her truth.

(Dip fingers, touch throat.)

Bless (name of the mother-to-be)'s heart

that she may open to the wisdom of all women.

(Dip fingers, touch heart.)

Bless (name of the mother-to-be)'s solar plexus

that she may live in the world in a way that is true to her

highest self.

(Dip fingers, touch solar plexus.)

Bless (name of the mother-to-be)'s belly

for the children or other creative gifts she has given.

(Dip fingers, touch navel.)

Bless (name of the mother-to-be's) vagina,

the gateway of birth.

(Dip fingers, touch pelvic bone.)

Bless (name of the mother-to-be)'s feet

that she may walk your divine path.

(Dip fingers, touch feet.)

Bless (name of the mother-to-be)'s hands

that do your work as well as her own.

(Dip fingers, touch hands.)

Bless (name of the mother-to-be), for she is your child:

a part of you, and a part of us all.

(Dip fingers, touch crown.)

CHAPTER 7

Ritual Stage 4: Completing

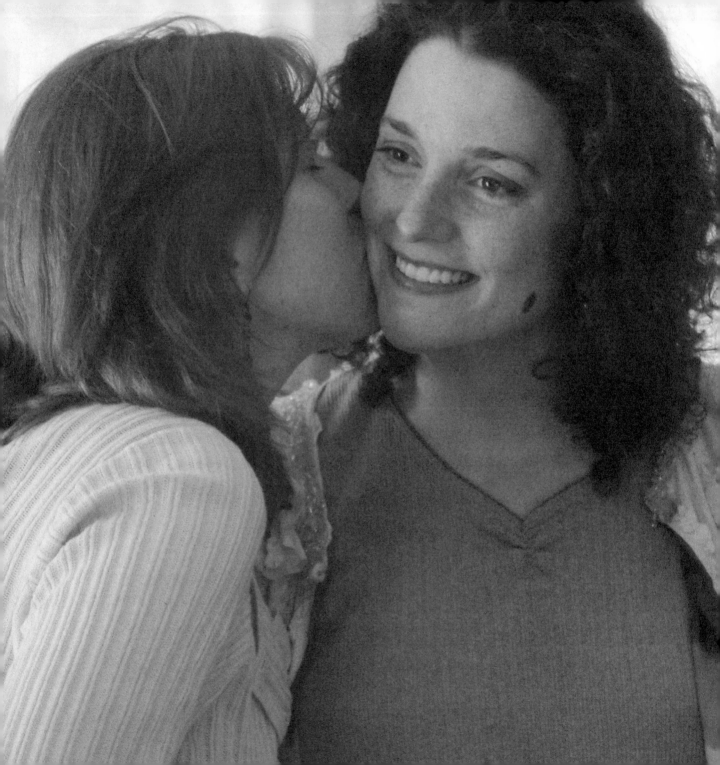

The Japanese heraldic emblem **Seed of the Universe**
is a symbol of potential energy.

BEFORE WE CAN BRING any ritual to a close, there are a couple of important things that need to happen. First, we need to raise energy specifically to concentrate the work we've done together in our circle, so that it may in turn be sent out into the ether in full force. Then we need to affirm our connection with the mother-to-be as well as with each other—weaving a web so these connections will continue beyond the blessingway event. And we need to thank God, Spirit, or any other energies that we have invited to join us during the course of the ritual; then we may open our sealed circle once again.

Raising Energy

Raising energy for the mother-to-be is a very important element of the blessingway. When you focus your attention on the work you have done during the course of the blessingway ritual, you can create warm, strong energy that flows through your bodies and your hearts—energy that is directly related to the discoveries made and the foundational work done together in your circle.

Raising energy makes your hopes, dreams, and intentions more tangible and real within the participants. When you succeed in doing this, you become charged with a power that glows outward from the women, even after leaving the blessingway circle.

WORKING WITH ENERGY

You can raise energy by having participants hold hands while engaging in one of the following activities:

- Sing or chant a powerful song
- Hum or tone (intone a particular sound together) to raise the energetic vibration
- Visualize or imagine your collective blessings, wishes, prayers, intentions, and affirmations forming a sphere or column of light
- Move together—hold hands and circle the central altar while steadily increasing your pace

This concentrated energy is sent out into the universe, where it is shared and empowered by all that is, and then returned to you. Choose one of the following options to send out the group energy:

- Listen and focus on the silence
- Feel the memory or vibration of the sound you created as it resonates within you
- Visualize the sphere or column of light you have imagined traveling upward
- Stop your movement, then raise your hands to the sky

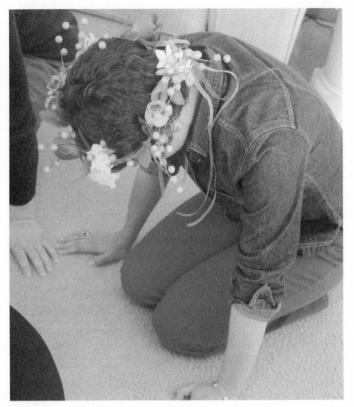

GUIDING ENERGY EFFECTIVELY

During the energy-raising segment of your ritual, someone will need to become the conductor of the group energy. Think of it as conducting an orchestra with your words and tone. Here is the score you will be following:

Build energy slowly: The chanting, visualizing, or moving will raise energy slowly and softly, but to be effective, it must build as it goes. Watch the group for signs of how the energy is going and, if need be, guide it to grow.

Bring the energy to a peak, then stop swiftly: When you feel the group energy has reached its crescendo, guide the group in releasing the energy to the world. To do this effectively, end the outpouring abruptly at its peak—before it begins to wane or dissipate—by stopping everyone in their tracks and having them immediately lift their arms up to the sky (while holding hands) in a big swooping motion.

Release the energy: Next, have everyone free their hands from one another and reach even higher, palms open, to send the energy up and outward to be shared. Guide the group to wait there for a few moments until the energy feels released.

When you receive the energy back, you need to ground it so any excess energy the circle cannot hold will be returned to the earth. Choose one of the following ways to ground the returning energy:

• Lay down or place your palms on the floor

• Consume a small portion of food

• Perform any action that serves to reconnect you to the physical or earth plane

Receive the energy back: Direct the group to open themselves to receive the energy—now enhanced by having been released and shared—back again.

Ground the excess energy: When the group feels that it has completely received the returning energy, invite the women to put their hands on the floor to ground any extra energy before moving on to the next part of the ritual.

Weaving a Web

Weaving a web of yarn is a very profound ritual element that is included in most blessingway rituals. The act of weaving a web enables you to stay connected to the mother-to-be beyond the day of the blessingway—through labor, birth, and on into her postpartum period. Weaving a web also symbolically reinforces your connection to each other, as well as to Spirit. We recommend wool yarn because it felts together and stays tied. Choose a color that supports your ritual's work, such as red to symbolize the color of life blood.

Begin the process of weaving a web by wrapping the tail end from a ball of yarn around one wrist several times, while explaining the web weaving process to the group. (The circle of women can be either seated or standing.) When you're done, toss the ball of yarn to a woman across from you, who will then wrap the yarn around her own wrist several times. This woman

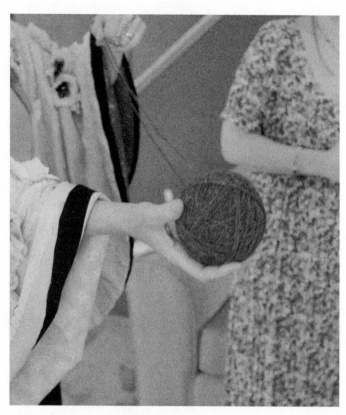

will toss the ball across the circle to another woman, who in turn will wrap her wrist. (Be sure to keep the yarn taut, but not tight, between the women.) After the last woman finishes, wrap the yarn around the Goddess candle on the central altar. (Leave a good deal of slack in the yarn that connects the circle of women to the candle.) Once the web has been completed, everyone should stand (if seated) and pull back slightly to feel the strength of the connections they

have just made. (Do this carefully so you don't topple over the Goddess candle.) Anchor this powerful experience by reciting Shekhinah Mountain-water's chant: *"We are the flow, we are the ebb, we are the weavers, we are the web."*

The final step of weaving your web involves scissors, so be sure they are close at hand before you start the whole process! You'll need to cut yourselves apart from one another, and then help each other tie

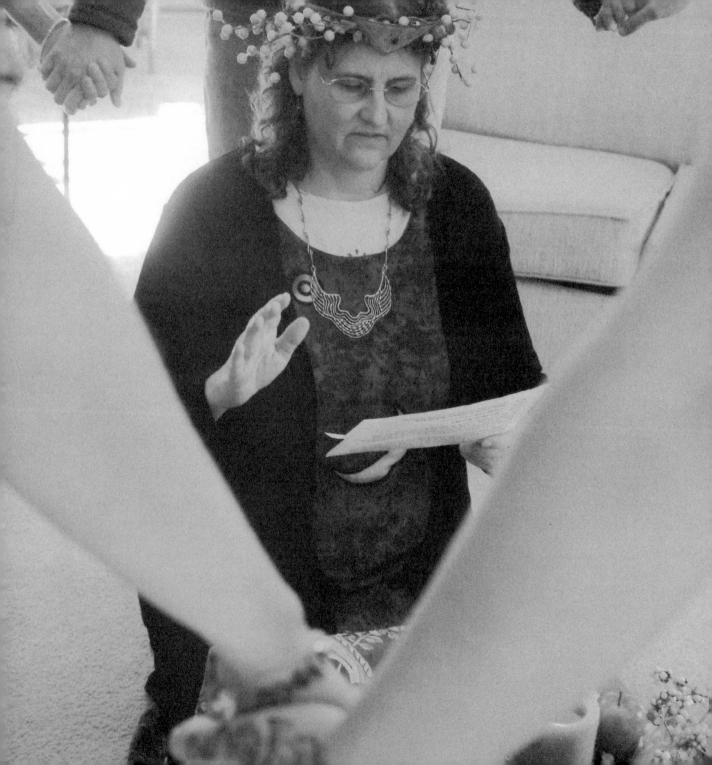

off the yarn on one another's wrists. (Secure the yarn around the Goddess candle as well.) This will effectively create a bracelet for each woman in the circle, each of whom should agree to wear their bracelet until after the baby has been born, or until the mom-to-be lets everyone know that her milk has come in and all is well.

Closing and Giving Thanks

To complete the blessingway ritual, you need to offer thanks to Spirit, the four directions, the Goddess, or whomever you invited into it. The following is an example of thanksgiving:

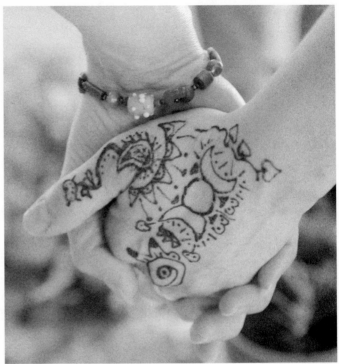

(Spirit), you have been an inspiration to all of us here today. We are grateful for your loving and powerful presence, and release you from this circle with our deepest thanks.

In support of the mother-to-be, you may wish to request that the Divine remain present with her—or with the entire circle—beyond the day of the blessingway event. The following is an example of giving thanks with an appeal for continued support:

(Spirit), we are grateful for your loving and powerful presence here with us today. We release you from this

circle with our thanks, asking that you remain with (name of the mother-to-be) from now until the birth of her baby.

When finished giving thanks, extinguish the Goddess candle on your central altar, then make a statement that acknowledges and anchors the value of your work, such as the following:

Today, we have succeeded in forming a beautiful, sacred space for (name of the mother-to-be)'s bless-

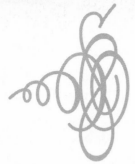
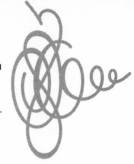

ingway. The strength and energy we have helped (name of the mother-to-be) to raise is shining inside her and radiating out for us all to see. The power of the feminine spirit has been unveiled in each of us today. May we carry the knowledge and gifts we've received on into everything we do from this day on. Let us stay connected to (name of the mother-to-be), creating a cradle of support, as she awaits her birthing day and beyond, as she learns to mother her new baby. This has been a powerful day.

At this point, check in with the mother-to-be to see how she's feeling and ensure that her needs have been met. When you have confirmed that your work is complete, open the circle and set out your feast.

Opening the Circle

When you cast your circle at the beginning of the blessingway, you created a container that cradled all of those working within it, as well as Spirit. You closed your circle around you at the beginning of the blessingway so all your work would stay safe, protected, and sacred. Now that your work has been completed, you need to open your circle back up again.

You can open a circle with a simple statement, such as "Our circle is now open, but remains unbroken." It's also nice to acknowledge the work that you have done—and do every day—before you leave and go your separate ways. There is a simple but powerful African prayer that can be recited to remind you of this:

Let us take care of our children, for they have a long way to go. Let us take care of our elders, for they have come a long way. Let us take care of those of us in between, for we are doing the work.

Additionally, there are many traditional songs and chants that work well to open a blessingway circle; "We Are a Circle within a Circle," "May the Circle Be Open," and "May the Long Time Sun" are just a few. (See page 137 for songbooks and musical recordings containing these and other wonderful chants.)

If you physically defined your circle at the beginning of your ritual, you will need to physically open it. Walk counterclockwise around the circle and, with a broom, sweep away the outline of the circle that you originally created by walking in a clockwise direction.

CHAPTER 8

Ritual Stage 5: Feasting

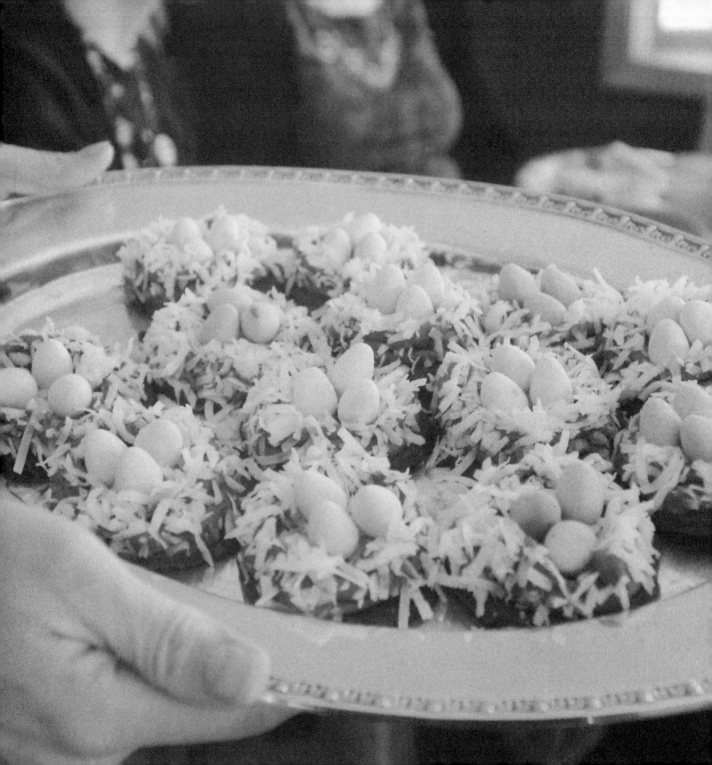

The **mandala** is a powerful symbol of the universe used by
many cultures. Its name is comprised from the root word *manda*
(essence), and the suffix *la* (container).

IT IS IMPORTANT TO INCLUDE A FEAST as part of every ritual because it supports our work in many significant ways. The feast celebrates the incredible degree to which the blessingway has brought us together. We build upon the excitement and appreciation of what we have all just experienced as we sit together—sharing sights, smells, and tastes as we partake in this very special meal.

Feasting smoothes our transition from sacred space back to the social space of our daily lives. We release any excess energy that may be left over from the ritual itself by filling our bodies with the bounty of Mother Earth, who grounds us. When we eat food, reawakening our connection to the earth, we bring our consciousness back into our physical selves. The experience of eating is itself heightened when included as part of a ritual. The simplest foods—bread, cheese, fruit—often taste exquisite.

When women eat together, serving each other scrumptious, lovingly prepared foods, we get the opportunity to show our mutual care and support. It is during the feast that we begin to normalize our blessingway experiences by revisiting them in an intimate, social setting—allowing them to become a part of our general life experience. The feast serves as a gateway, and together we pass through it, linking our ritual life with the path we walk each day.

This is an especially good time to give thanks, not only for our meal and our friendships, but for all the time, energy, and effort the women present put into organizing, leading, and participating in the blessingway event. While everyone is chatting and enjoying the meal, we can make announcements, pass out copies of the phone tree, distribute labor candles, string the mom-to-be's blessingway bracelet, put the finishing touches on other collective gifts, or even swap recipes.

Our Collection of Recipes

Recipes can be kept hidden away like coveted secrets, creating boundaries between us. Or they can given freely as offerings of love and friendship. In this spirit, we'd like to share some of our favorite blessingway feast recipes with you.

❀ · ❀ · ❀ · ❀ · ❀

Raspberry Cream Cheese Coffee Cake

[Serves 8]

Because of its rich and creamy center, eating this coffee cake is a sensual experience!

For cake batter:

2¼ cups all-purpose flour

¾ cup sugar

¾ cup butter, chilled

½ teaspoon baking powder

½ teaspoon baking soda

¼ teaspoon salt

¾ cup sour cream

1 teaspoon almond or vanilla extract

1 egg

For filling:

1 (8-ounce) package cream cheese, softened

¼ cup sugar

1 egg

For toppings:

½ cup raspberry preserves

½ cup sliced almonds

Preheat oven to 350°F.

Grease and flour the bottom and sides of a 9- or 10-inch springform pan.

In a large bowl, combine flour and ¾ cup sugar; mix well. With a pastry blender or a fork, cut in butter until mixture resembles coarse crumbs. Reserve 1 cup of crumb mixture.

To remaining crumb mixture, add baking powder, baking soda, salt, sour cream, almond or vanilla extract, and 1 egg. Blend well. Spread batter about ¼ inch thick over bottom and 2 inches up sides of greased and floured pan.

In a small bowl, combine cream cheese, ¼ cup sugar, and 1 egg. Blend well. Pour filling into the batter-lined pan. Carefully spoon preserves evenly over the cream cheese mixture.

In another small bowl, combine reserved crumb mixture and sliced almonds, then sprinkle over the preserves.

Bake for 45 to 55 minutes or until cream cheese filling is set and the crust is a deep golden brown. Cool 15 minutes and then remove the sides of the pan.

❀ . ❀ . ❀ . ❀ . ❀

Carrot-Raisin Muffins

[Makes 1 dozen]

Just as yummy as carrot cake!

2 cups all-purpose flour
1 cup sugar
2 teaspoons baking powder
¼ teaspoon ginger
½ teaspoon cinnamon
½ cup raisins
½ cup walnuts, chopped
½ cup carrots, grated
1 (8-ounce) can crushed pineapple, undrained
2 eggs, beaten
½ cup butter, melted, or ½ cup vegetable oil
1 teaspoon vanilla extract

Preheat oven to 375°F.

Sift together flour, sugar, baking powder, ginger, and cinnamon into a large mixing bowl. Stir in raisins, walnuts, carrot, pineapple with juice, eggs, butter, and vanilla. Mix thoroughly. Pour into a greased or paper-lined muffin pan. Bake for 20 to 25 minutes.

❀ . ❀ . ❀ . ❀ . ❀

Sesame Eggplant Salsa with Parmesan Pita Crisps

[Makes about 4 cups]

This Asian-influenced vegan dip delivers a spicy kick.

2 medium eggplants
1 tablespoon vegetable or peanut oil
¾ cup packed minced green onions, plus extra
   for garnish
2½ tablespoons fresh ginger, peeled and minced
4 garlic cloves, minced
1 teaspoon chile-garlic sauce
3 tablespoons packed golden brown sugar
2 tablespoons soy sauce
1 tablespoon rice vinegar
2 teaspoons fresh lemon juice
2 large plum tomatoes, seeded and chopped
¾ cup packed fresh cilantro, finely chopped, plus
   extra for garnish
1½ teaspoons sesame oil

Preheat oven to 425°F.

Pierce eggplants all over with a fork. Place on a baking sheet. Roast in the oven until eggplants are very soft and deflated, turning once, about 1 hour. Cool slightly. Cut eggplants in half; scrape the flesh into a strainer set over a large bowl (do not allow bottom of strainer to touch bowl). Let eggplant drain 30 minutes. Transfer eggplant to a food processor; process by pulsing until almost smooth.

Heat vegetable oil in large, heavy skillet over medium-high heat. Add ¾ cup green onions, ginger, garlic, and chile-garlic sauce; sauté just until onions soften, about 1 minute. Stir in brown sugar, soy sauce, rice vinegar, and lemon juice. Bring to simmer, stirring constantly.

Mix in eggplant purée and cook until heated through, about 2 minutes. Remove from heat. Stir in tomatoes, ¾ cup cilantro, and sesame oil. Cool to room temperature. Season with salt and pepper. Transfer to a medium bowl. Garnish eggplant salsa with 1 tablespoon each green onions and cilantro. Serve with Parmesan Pita Crisps.

❀ . ❀ . ❀ . ❀ . ❀

Parmesan Pita Crisps
[Makes 6 dozen]

6 (6-inch-diameter) pita breads (white or wheat)
6 tablespoons olive oil
1¼ cups freshly grated Parmesan cheese
Black pepper

Preheat oven to 375°F.

Cut each pita bread horizontally in half, forming 2 pita disks. Brush inside of disks with olive oil. Sprinkle disks with Parmesan cheese, then pepper.

Cut each disk into 6 wedges. Arrange pita wedges in single layer on a large baking sheet. Bake until pita wedges are golden and just crisp, about 12 minutes.

Cook's note: Can be prepared 3 days ahead. Cool completely, then store in an airtight container at room temperature. Rewarm in 325°F oven for 5 minutes.

❀ . ❀ . ❀ . ❀ . ❀

Snack Mix
[Makes about 10 to 12 cups]
We make this snack mix to pass around a blessingway circle for quick energy. It makes a wonderful postpartum snack for nursing mothers, too.

Nuts (peanuts, almonds, cashews, peanuts, soy)
Sesame sticks
Yogurt-covered raisins
Pretzels (plain, yogurt-covered, peanut butter–covered)
Dried fruit (cranberries, raisins, apricots, apples)
Seeds (pumpkin, sunflower)
Banana chips
Coconut
Carob chips
Chocolate-covered cherries
Chocolate-covered espresso beans
M&Ms

Use about a cup each of whichever ingredients you choose to include from our list. Try different combinations of ingredients, experimenting with roasted/raw, salted/unsalted, chocolate/nonchocolate, and healthy/nonhealthy items. Whatever you mix up will be yummy.

❀ · ❀ · ❀ · ❀ · ❀

Tamale Pie

[Serves 8]

This spicy dish can be easily made ahead of time, then reheated. It also makes a hearty postpartum meal.

For filling:

2 tablespoons olive oil
1 medium onion, chopped
1 green bell pepper, chopped
2 garlic cloves, minced
1 pound ground turkey or soy substitute
2 tablespoons chili powder
1½ teaspoons dried oregano
1 teaspoon ground cumin
¼ teaspoon cayenne pepper
½ teaspoon salt
1 (28-ounce) can peeled tomatoes, drained,
   coarsely chopped
1 (15-ounce) can tomato sauce
1 (15-ounce) can black beans
1 (6-ounce) can pitted black olives, sliced
1 (15-ounce) can whole kernel corn

For topping:

4 cups water
2 teaspoons salt
2 cups yellow corn meal or polenta
2 to 3 cups grated Monterey Jack or cheddar cheese

Preheat oven to 375°F.

In a large, deep skillet, heat the oil. Add the onion, green pepper, and garlic. Cook over medium heat, stirring often, until the vegetables are softened, about 3 minutes. Add the ground turkey (or soy substitute) and cook, stirring and breaking up the meat with a wooden spoon, until the turkey loses its pink color, about 3 minutes. (The soy substitute does not have to cook; it just needs to be broken up.)

Add the chili powder, oregano, cumin, cayenne, and ½ teaspoon of salt. Cook, stirring, for 1 minute. Add the tomatoes, tomato sauce, black beans, olives, and corn. Bring to a boil, reduce heat to medium-low, and simmer until the filling is thickened, 15 to 20 minutes. Spoon the filling into a 9 by 13-inch baking dish, spreading evenly.

In a large saucepan, bring the water and 2 teaspoons of salt to a boil over high heat. Gradually whisk in the cornmeal, reduce the heat to low, and cook, whisking constantly, until thickened and all water is absorbed (about 1 or 2 minutes). Spread the warm cornmeal topping over the filling. (The tamale pie can be prepared to this point up to 1 day ahead, then covered and refrigerated.)

Bake for 30 minutes (40 minutes if refrigerated). Sprinkle the grated cheese over the top and continue baking until the cheese is melted, about 10 minutes more.

Cook's note: Can reheat at 375°F for about 30 minutes, or until cheese is bubbling.

❀ · ❀ · ❀ · ❀ · ❀

Ham-and-Spinach Bread Pudding

[Serves 8]

Impressive and well worth taking the time to make, this is a great brunch or dinner meal.

2 large baguettes
4 tablespoons unsalted butter, melted
2 onions, chopped
2 tablespoons olive oil
1 pound cooked ham, cut into ½-inch cubes
4 large eggs
1 quart whole milk
1 teaspoon salt
¼ teaspoon nutmeg
Ground black pepper
6 cups spinach leaves (about 1 bunch), coarsely chopped
1 pound Fontina cheese, grated

Preheat broiler.

Diagonally cut baguettes crosswise into ¾-inch-thick slices, and brush both sides with melted butter. Toast on a baking sheet under the broiler, 3 inches from the heat, until golden, about 30 seconds on each side.

Preheat oven to 350°F.

Sauté onions in oil in a 12-inch nonstick skillet over medium-high heat, stirring occasionally, until golden. Add ham and sauté, stirring occasionally, until ham is lightly browned.

Whisk eggs in a large bowl, then whisk in milk, salt, nutmeg, and pepper to taste. Add the toasted bread and toss gently. Transfer the saturated bread to a shallow 3-quart casserole dish, slightly overlapping slices. Add any remaining egg mixture.

Tuck spinach and ham between the bread slices, reserving a little ham to sprinkle over the top. Sprinkle cheese over the pudding, lifting bread slices with a spatula to allow some cheese to fall between them. Sprinkle the reserved ham over the pudding, and bake in the middle of the oven for 45 minutes to 1 hour, or until puffed and the edges of the bread are golden and the custard is set in the middle.

Cook's note: Do not overcook or the custard will become watery! Check carefully at 45 minutes; it rarely needs to cook any longer. This bread pudding can be assembled one day ahead and then chilled, covered. Increase baking time to 1 hour and 15 minutes if the bread pudding is cold when put into the oven. Cover the top with foil after 45 minutes to prevent overbrowning.

❀ · ❀ · ❀ · ❀ · ❀

African Vegetable Stew

[Serves 4]

Tasty and easy to make, this is an earthy one-pot dish.

1 large bunch Swiss chard
1 large onion, chopped
1 clove garlic, chopped
2 tablespoons vegetable oil
1 (15-ounce) can chickpeas, drained, rinsed
½ cup raisins
2 yams, peeled and sliced into ½-inch-thick slabs
1 (28-ounce) can whole peeled tomatoes (or 3 to 4 large, fresh tomatoes)
1 teaspoon salt
1 teaspoon black pepper
½ cup raw white rice
Tabasco sauce

Wash and destem Swiss chard. Chop the stems and place in a large stew pot. Chop the leaves and set aside. Fry the Swiss chard stems, onion, and garlic in oil until the chard is fairly limp. Add the chopped leaves and fry a bit longer. Next add chickpeas, raisins, yams, tomatoes (with juice), salt, and pepper. Cook a couple of minutes.

Make a well in the center of the mixture in the pot. Put the rice in the well, and pat it down until it is wet. Cover and cook until the rice is done, about 25 minutes. Add Tabasco sauce to taste.

Cook's note: This recipe is difficult to double, since everything cooks in one pot. When we have tried to double it, the rice did not cook completely—so when we need a lot of this stew, we make several batches, using separate pots.

❀ · ❀ · ❀ · ❀ · ❀

Carrot-Ginger Soup and Irish Soda Bread

[Serves 4]

This simple root vegetable soup, served with a warm loaf of Irish Soda Bread, makes a perfect postpartum meal on a crisp autumn day. Double this recipe for potlucks.

1½ cups chopped onions
1½ tablespoons peeled and grated ginger
1 tablespoon vegetable oil
4 cups sliced carrots
4 cups vegetable or chicken stock
2 teaspoons salt
½ cup milk, cream, or soy milk
1 teaspoon pepper

Sauté onions together with the ginger and oil in a large soup pot until they are soft and golden. Add carrots, stock, and salt. Bring to a boil, then reduce to a simmer and cook about 40 minutes. Remove from the heat and add milk, cream, or soy milk. Using a food processor or blender, purée the soup. Return the soup to the pot to reheat, and add pepper.

❀ . ❀ . ❀ . ❀ . ❀

Irish Soda Bread

[Makes 1 round loaf]

This beautiful and fragrant bread is so simple you can have it baking in about 10 minutes.

2 cups all-purpose flour
2 cups whole-wheat flour
½ cup sugar
2 teaspoons baking soda
1 teaspoon salt
4 tablespoons butter, chilled
1 cup raisins
1½ cups buttermilk or plain yogurt

Preheat oven to 350°F.

In a bowl, combine dry ingredients. Cut in the butter until it is pea sized (by hand or with a food processor). Stir in the raisins and buttermilk (or yogurt). Turn the dough onto a floured surface and knead 1 minute, then shape into a disk about 8 inches in diameter. Cut an X into the top and bake on a greased baking sheet for 45 to 50 minutes.

❀ . ❀ . ❀ . ❀ . ❀

Sumi Salad

[Serves 12]

This salad can easily be made the night before and stored in the refrigerator.

For dressing:

¼ cup soy sauce
¼ cup honey
¾ cup vegetable oil
6 tablespoons rice vinegar
1 teaspoon black pepper
1 teaspoon salt

For salad:

¼ cup almonds, slivered
¼ cup sesame seeds
2 packages ramen noodles
8 scallions, chopped
1 head of Chinese (napa) cabbage, finely chopped
2 cups snow peas
2 cups mung bean sprouts

In a jar with a lid, combine the dressing ingredients. Shake and set aside.

Toast the almonds and sesame seeds in the oven or toaster oven until light brown. Break up the ramen noodles while still in the package, then cook as directed. (Do not add the seasoning packet.) As soon as the noodles are done, rinse them in a strainer under cold water. Place in a large bowl together with the toasted almonds and sesame seeds. Add the scallions, cabbage, snow peas, and bean sprouts. Shake the dressing again, then add to the salad.

❁ . ❁ . ❁ . ❁ . ❁

Lemon Pasta Salad with Feta Cheese

[Serves 8]

Very simple, very tasty. The toasted pine nuts and parsley round out the flavors in this lemony salad.

For dressing:

7 tablespoons extra-virgin olive oil
4 tablespoons fresh lemon juice
3 tablespoons whole-grain mustard
2 garlic cloves, minced
2 teaspoons lemon peel, grated

For salad:

12 ounces penne pasta
2 cups small cherry tomatoes, halved
1½ cups chopped red bell pepper
1½ cups crumbled feta cheese
1 cup chopped green onions
¼ cup finely chopped parsley
1 cup pine nuts, toasted

Whisk oil, lemon juice, mustard, garlic, and lemon peel in a small bowl to blend. Season dressing with salt and pepper.

Cook the penne in a large pot of boiling salted water until tender but still firm to bite. Drain the pasta, rinse with cold water to cool it quickly, and then drain again. Transfer the pasta to a large bowl. Add tomatoes, bell pepper, feta cheese, green onions, parsley, and pine nuts. Pour the dressing over the salad and toss to coat. Season to taste with salt and pepper.

Variation: Try using finely chopped mint in place of the parsley, or a combination of the two, for a variation of this pasta salad.

❁ . ❁ . ❁ . ❁ . ❁

Oatmeal Nursing Cookies

[Makes 4 dozen]

Cookies make great snacks for nursing mothers, especially when the cookies are packed with lots of healthy ingredients. Consider delivering a freshly baked batch as part of a new mom's postpartum meal.

1 cup raisins
1 cup butter, melted
1 teaspoon vanilla
3 eggs
1 cup packed brown sugar
1 cup granulated sugar
2½ cups all-purpose flour
1 teaspoon salt
1 teaspoon cinnamon
2 teaspoons baking soda
1½ cups rolled oats
½ cup wheat germ
¾ cup pecans, chopped
1 cup chocolate chips (optional)

Preheat oven to 350°F.

In the bowl of an electric mixer, soak raisins in melted butter and vanilla for 1 hour. Add eggs and sugars; beat well.

In a separate bowl, combine flour, salt, cinnamon, baking soda, oats, and wheat germ. Slowly add the dry mixture to the wet. Stir in the pecans and chocolate chips by hand. Spoon onto greased baking sheets. Bake for 10 to 12 minutes.

❀ · ❀ · ❀ · ❀ · ❀

Molasses Postpartum Cookies
[Makes 5 dozen]
Another nutritious, easy-to-eat snack, these cookies contain iron-rich molasses (new moms can become depleted in iron due to blood loss) and apricots to help regulate bowel function. A little love and nurturing in every bite!

1 cup granulated sugar
½ cup packed brown sugar
1 cup butter, softened
1 large egg
½ cup molasses
2¼ cups all-purpose flour
2 teaspoons ground ginger
½ teaspoon ground allspice
1 teaspoon cinnamon
2 teaspoons baking soda
½ teaspoon salt
¼ teaspoon ground white pepper
1 cup finely chopped apricots (optional)

Preheat oven to 350°F.
Put ½ cup of the granulated sugar, all of the brown sugar, and the butter in the bowl of an electric mixer.

Cream the butter and sugars on medium speed for 2 minutes, until the mixture is light and fluffy. Continue mixing. Add egg, then molasses.

Sift the dry ingredients together and add to wet mixture; mix well using low speed. Stir in the apricots by hand. Refrigerate the dough for 30 minutes.

Form the dough into 1-inch balls, and roll them in the remaining granulated sugar. Place cookies 2 to 3 inches apart on two greased baking sheets. Flatten them slightly with your fingers.

Bake the cookies about 12 minutes, until golden brown and set around the edges but still soft inside. Let them cool 5 minutes, and then remove from the baking sheets to a wire rack to cool.

❀ · ❀ · ❀ · ❀ · ❀

Bird's Nest Cookies

[Makes 2 dozen]

These cookies are especially fun to make for blessingways since they symbolize birth and new life.

1 cup butter, softened
½ cup plus 2 tablespoons sugar
1¾ cups all-purpose flour, plus more for rolling out
    dough
¼ teaspoon salt
½ cup Dutch-process cocoa powder
6 ounces semisweet chocolate, chopped, or
    chocolate chips
1 cup heavy cream
1 teaspoon instant espresso powder
2 cups shredded sweetened coconut
6 to 8 dozen candy-coated chocolate eggs (we use
    Cadbury's mini eggs; they look the most realistic)

Preheat oven to 350°F.

Grease (or line with parchment paper) two baking sheets. In the bowl of an electric mixer, combine butter and sugar. In a separate bowl, sift together flour, salt, and cocoa powder. Add the flour mixture to the butter mixture, and beat on low until a stiff dough forms, about 2 minutes. Transfer the dough to a piece of plastic wrap, wrap tightly, and chill until firm, about 30 minutes.

Meanwhile, place the chocolate, heavy cream, and espresso powder in a medium-sized heat-proof bowl. Place the bowl over a pan of gently simmering water, stirring occasionally, until the chocolate melts, creating a ganache. Remove the bowl from the heat, and set the chocolate ganache aside to cool, stirring occasionally.

On a lightly floured surface, roll out the chilled dough to a ¼-inch thickness. Using a 2¼-inch round cookie cutter, cut out 24 cookies, and place them on the baking sheets. Chill the cookies until firm, about 20 minutes.

Bake the cookies until set, about 14 minutes. Carefully transfer to a wire rack to cool.

When the ganache has cooled to room temperature, whisk it until it becomes stiff enough to pipe. Transfer the ganache to a pastry bag fitted with a ⅜-inch round tip. Pipe the ganache around the perimeter of the cookies to create the sides of a nest. Sprinkle coconut onto the ganache, and then turn each cookie upside down to remove excess coconut. Fill each nest with 3 or 4 chocolate eggs.

❀ · ❀ · ❀ · ❀ · ❀

Mint Lemonade

[Serves 8]

We like to leave the mint in our lemonade, but you can strain it out if you chop it more coarsely. Just refrigerate the drink (with the mint) for an hour or two before straining, so the mint flavor will infuse the lemonade.

½ to ¾ cup mint leaves
1½ cups sugar
7 cups water
2 cups lemon juice
Mint sprigs for garnish

Place the mint leaves in a food processor and pulse until finely chopped. Add sugar ½ cup at a time and process until well blended. Combine the water and lemon juice in a pitcher, then add mint sugar. Stir until thoroughly mixed. Serve over ice and garnish with a mint sprig.

❀ · ❀ · ❀ · ❀ · ❀

Mother's Blessing Tea

[Makes several quarts]

Angela Tiberio, the owner of our local herb shop Lavender Moon, developed this healing tea. Brew it for a new mom to drink right after delivery and during the days following birth. It soothes the nervous system, reduces stress, helps muscles to recover from labor, encourages milk flow, and aids digestion.

1 ounce red raspberry leaf
1 ounce catnip
1 ounce chamomile
½ ounce fennel seed
1 ounce nettle
¼ ounce rose petals
¼ ounce cinnamon chips (¼-inch pieces) or
    ½ cinnamon stick

By the quart:
Combine the herbs. Put 4 tablespoons of the mixture in a quart glass jar, fill with boiling water, cover, then steep for 20 minutes.

By the cup:
Combine the herbs. Place 2 heaping teaspoons of the mixture in a tea ball, place in a cup, cover with boiling water, then steep for 20 minutes.

CHAPTER 9

Leading a Blessingway

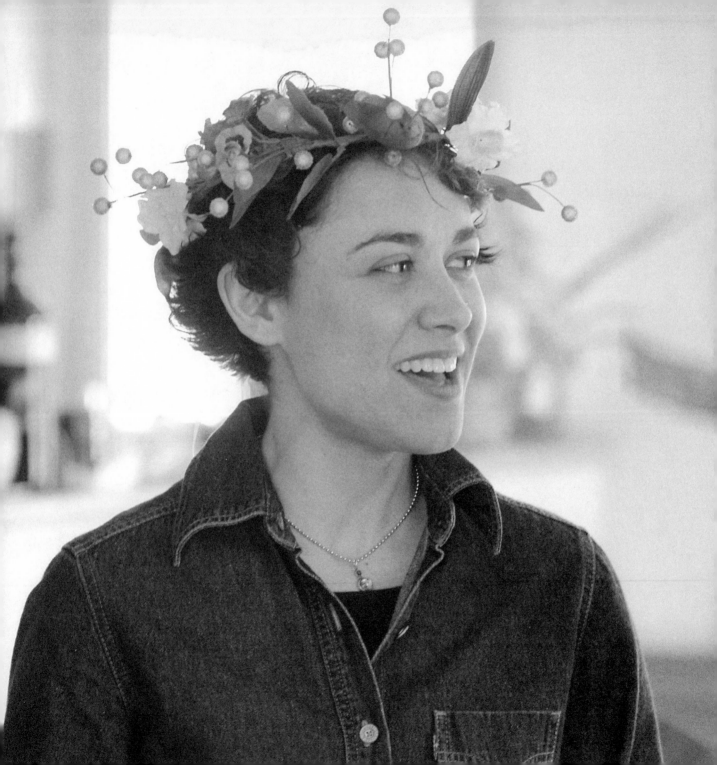

A sacred geometric symbol, the universal **Flower of Life** shows the
connectedness of all things and the oneness of life.

THE BLESSINGWAY FACILITATOR guides the circle
of women's energy and emotion to achieve the greatest enjoyment and deepest blessingway experience.
Knowing the ritual elements well, she first plants the
seeds of intention, then she cultivates these seeds as
she leads the women through the ritual outline in a
way that establishes safety, draws out wisdom, unveils
power, and fills hearts with great joy and beauty.

Getting Ready for the Ritual

As the blessingway facilitator or leader, one of the
most helpful tools you can prepare for yourself is a facilitator's copy of the blessingway outline. Your copy
of the outline can be as general or as specific as you
like, though ideally it should include all the information you'll need to lead the ritual. Depending upon
the complexity of your blessingway, include details
such as the time estimates for each section, the name
of the woman leading each section, verbal and visual
cues throughout, logistical reminders, or any instructions you'll need to guide the circle of women.

The first part of a facilitator's outline looks something like this:

❀ · ❀ · ❀ · ❀ · ❀
Johanna's Blessingway

Welcome (Donna, 10:00–10:10)
Donna reads her prepared statement.

Smudging (Yana, 10:10–10:20)
Barb starts music: "Tierra Mi Cuerpo" by Beverly
Frederick (Tracks 1–10 on CD, approx.12 minutes)

Yana gives a brief introduction to the practice of
smudging, and she invites the women to line up from
oldest to youngest outside on the porch. As each one
steps up, she says: "Take a deep breath, relax, and let
the smoke from the burning sage carry away all that
is not needed here today."

REHEARSING

Schedule at least one rehearsal prior to the day of the
blessingway. Invite all the women who will be leading
segments or coordinating activities during the event.
Talk through the ritual, then walk through the ritual,
because what works on paper doesn't always work in
real life (for example, if you are reading a poem on
motherhood at the beginning of the pampering segment, make sure that someone else is preparing the

Guiding Meditations Effectively

When guiding a group through a meditation or visualization, keep these points in mind:

Tone: Allow your voice to be steady and rich, and speak slowly.

Pace: Take some time in the beginning of your meditation to help the circle feel relaxed. Deep breaths are good. Bring the women's attention to their body parts. Guide them to release tension by using deep breaths and the power of their minds. Have them focus on their breath, and then take them on a trip.

Pauses: Give the women time to experience the journey and to sense what they need to sense. (In other words, pause.) Once you have chosen or written your meditation, practice it by reading it to yourself to determine how long it takes you to move through each part of the meditation. Be sure to note your pauses in parentheses.

Focus: Trust yourself to know how fast or slow to go by opening your heart to the circle of women. With your written notes as guidelines, use your senses to tell you when it's actually time to move on. Think of it as turning on your radar!

Closing: After the journey is completed, bring the women gently back to the present. Invite them to take their time returning. Guide them to gradually become aware of their bodies again, and then to open their eyes very slowly when they feel ready, allowing ample time for their eyes to readjust to the light in the room.

even breaks will help even out the ritual flow.

Guided meditations should be read all the way through during rehearsal, as if you're really at the ceremony. Ask others present to close their eyes and follow along. Read slowly and loudly, and include all pauses. If you will be playing music in the background during the ritual, be sure that the length of your selection runs about ten minutes longer than your meditation. You can always cue someone to fade the music down as your meditation comes to completion, but it can be very disruptive if the music halts before the meditation ends.

PREPARING THE SITE

Before you actually begin any ritual, you first have to set the stage to do your work. This is done by defining the specific area or ritual space where you will be forming your circle. The space itself should be delineated in some way from the rest of the house or area in which you will be casually gathering. Make your ritual area look special, so when the women enter it to form the blessingway circle, they will feel its difference.

Furniture should be arranged in as close to a circle formation as possible, with the mother-to-be's seat

mother-to-be's footbath). As you work your way through your blessingway outline, pay particular attention to the transition between ritual segments. If any are awkward or too abrupt, readings, poems, or

placed in a prominent position. If the circle of women will be sitting on the floor, your central altar should be on the floor as well, so it doesn't prevent the women from seeing one another. If you will be seated on chairs or couches, a coffee table (or other low table) can be used to create the central altar. TV tray tables make great altars for the four directions since they are small, uniform in size, and can be easily set about a room. Supplies should be placed near the area where you will be using them, but not in a way that clutters the ritual space. Make sure that all segment leaders know where their supplies are—they may even want to keep them under their seats.

It's important to clear the atmosphere or energy of the house (or space) in which you are gathering. A good way to do this is by walking through the ritual space in a counterclockwise direction while ringing bells or smudging. This "backward" movement will in effect "unwind" and release old energies. You can reset the energy and tone for the space as part of your ritual, or you can do it before the women arrive, by moving through the space or rooms in the reverse, clockwise direction while blessing it with prayers, sprinkling water, or ringing bells.

It will take you at least a couple of hours to fully prepare the space and yourself on the day of the event. (Ideally, the mother-to-be should do as little work as possible, so if the blessingway is to be held at

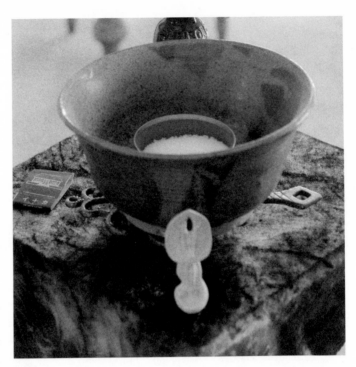

her home, please offer to come over the day before if any general cleaning is needed.) Be sure you plan enough time for setup, as you don't want to create a hectic atmosphere by rushing to finish preparations as the guests start to arrive.

PREPARING YOURSELF

As the ritual leader, it's important to take time to center yourself before attempting to guide others through the blessingway experience. Before beginning the blessingway, take some time to breathe deeply, quiet your mind, and open yourself wide so

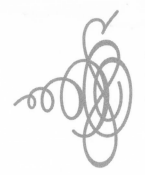
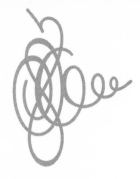

WE CAN BECOME SKILLED AT ALLOWING THE
WORLD IN, TAKING ITS SECRETS TO HEART,
AND FINDING POWER OUTSIDE OF OURSELVES.

—Thomas Moore, *The Education of the Heart*

the energy of Spirit may flow freely through you.

It's a good idea to request that any participants who will be leading ritual segments arrive early on the day of the blessingway. Meet briefly with each leader during set-up time to gain a sense of her energy. Offer your confidence, support, and encouragement. Remind all leaders to breathe, and ask that they speak slowly and at a volume that all in the circle will be able to hear. Then invite them to join you in the following pre-blessingway centering ritual:

Connect to Spirit: Sit in a circle around an unlit candle. Say a prayer of your own, or read the following invocation aloud, then light the candle. "(God/Goddess/Spirit), with the lighting of this candle we ask that you be with us today as we help prepare (name of the mother-to-be) for her journey to motherhood. Please let us act as conduits for your work, and may everything we do and say at this blessingway be inspired by you."

Put away concerns and distractions: Write down any concerns that you perceive could affect your ability to stay present and focused while you are leading the blessingway. For example: "I place my nervousness (my need to be perfect, my ego, my personal agenda, my concern that my children may miss me) in this container for safe keeping during this ritual." Fold the paper up and place in a safe, covered container (a jar or box) for the duration of the ritual.

Meditate: Take five to ten minutes for a silent, guided, or music meditation. Focus on your breath to become centered and relaxed.

Determine a focal point: Look around the room, or even out the window, to find an object to connect with. It should be something that brings forth your inner strength when you look at it (such as a strong tree outside or an inspirational piece of artwork on the wall). Spend some time focusing on the object and know that you may draw your attention to it anytime during the blessingway to gain strength, guidance, or help with letting go.

Let go: Remind yourself that you are merely a conduit for Spirit to work through, and once all the blessingway preparations have been completed, the ritual is really out of your hands. Your job now is to remain in conscious contact with Spirit, and to allow the divine plan to unfold.

Guiding the Blessingway Circle

One of your primary goals as the ritual leader will be to maintain the circle's safety and integrity. A blessingway circle often includes several women who are pregnant or nursing infants, so for this reason, you'll need to make space for these women to take care

related to her upcoming task

of their needs during the ritual. Nevertheless, it is disruptive to the circle's energy if the women are frequently moving in and out. To minimize disruption, ask the women to limit their comings and goings, and to maintain ritual silence any time they need to leave the circle. Additionally, make a pitcher of water and glasses available to be passed to anyone who needs a drink during the ritual. Place several small bowls with seeds, nuts, and dried fruits around the circle so the women may keep their energy levels up without leaving. (See chapter 8 for a nourishing snack mix recipe.)

SETTING THE TONE

A ritual leader guides the group of women's energy and emotion toward the greatest enjoyment and deepest experience of the ritual. Blessingways are by design made up of both serious and joyful activities. (Releasing fear is very intense, while pampering and adorning is lighthearted and fun.) One way to guide the participants effectively is by introducing, or setting the tone for, each segment of the ritual. Letting the women know what they will be doing and why they will be doing it will help them rise to the occasion.

When introducing a ritual segment, resist the temptation to simply say, *"And now we're going to pamper Donna."* Though straight to the point, this doesn't set the appropriate tone for the activity, nor will it evoke the feelings of great care and gentle nurturing that are essential to this central element of a blessingway. Your introduction should be more like the following:

The pathway to birth is a journey of a lifetime. We have gathered together today to help prepare Donna to make this journey. If everyone will move in closer to Donna, we can begin. Donna, we will be brushing your hair to untangle any snarls and to straighten out anything that's left undone, in order to ensure a smooth labor. We will be massaging your shoulders to help prepare you for bearing the responsibilities of motherhood. We will massage your hands to ready them for the physically hard work of motherhood. And we will bathe your feet to soothe them and clear the way for a peaceful journey.

If the blessingway is a new experience for anyone in the circle you're guiding, invite someone to start an activity—such as releasing fear—whom you know is familiar with ritual, or at least will feel comfortable carrying out the requested task. In some cases, you may be the best choice to model the appropriate manner of participating.

READING AND GUIDING GROUP ENERGY

Paying attention to how your personal power, as well as the circle's collective power, is flowing throughout a ritual will truly help everyone open to the experience. Power can be raised up or quieted down by different actions. Dancing raises power and energy levels. Quiet readings and meditations calm power and lower energy levels. As the facilitator, you can use your power to shift the circle's attention away from distractions, and to ground the women firmly in the ideas and activities that support the blessingway journey.

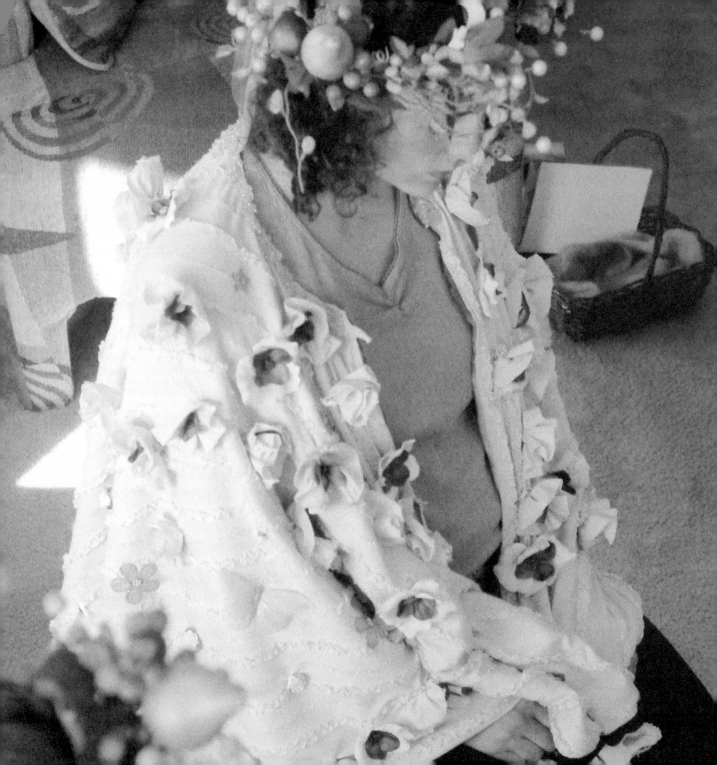

But what if you find that the circle of women isn't ready to come along? (In fact, one woman giggled through a meditation…several others refused to sing a chant…and still another woman denied having any fears to release.) First, take a deep breath. Then, as you let it out, remember that as the ritual leader, you have the power to shift the energy of a difficult group!

Exploring and growing are not always easy, so here are four techniques to use when faced with challenging circumstances:

Breathe and let go: It's possible that the issues that are coming up for certain women are just what they need to experience before they can fully participate in the ritual. Also realize that some women may not manage to get through their blocks during their time with you, so don't attach yourself to their behavior.

Be supportive: Offering your support may give some women the permission they need to speak truthfully about what is bubbling up. If not, trust that whatever feels difficult is probably a chance for everyone in the room to practice something that needs practicing, such as patience, kindness, or letting go.

Offer guidance: You can always approach someone by trying to give them words, but be sure to guide with compassion, for each person processes differently and grows only when they are ready. "This is hard for you, isn't it? Shall we take a break and regroup in five minutes?"

Check in: If you feel sure that things have really gotten too far off track, call for a break, then privately check in with the mother-to-be to determine how she's feeling. Or meet with the other leaders to discuss the best course of action.

KEEPING TIME

The ritual facilitator is theoretically responsible for keeping an eye on things and maintaining the ritual flow. However, it is also your goal to remain flexible, so if anything important or unexpected comes up, you can make time for it (while still being mindful of the ritual objectives and overall timing). Your job will be much easier in this regard if the ritual has been designed with this in mind, and not overcrowded with ritual elements or activities.

To help gauge how well you're staying on schedule throughout the blessingway, include the actual time you have estimated for each segment on your facilitator's outline and check it periodically. What if you got started a bit late, introductions took longer than you anticipated, or a guest shared a beautiful, touching, relevant (but unexpected) story? Whatever has occurred—you're now behind schedule. Don't panic; you can make up for lost time by combining ritual elements. You will find you have many opportunities to do this, such as: sharing altar items during personal introductions, presenting gifts while pampering the mother-to-be, or offering blessings while weaving the web.

Another way to stay on schedule is to shift a planned activity that can be accomplished after the ritual. Creating birth art, stringing beads, putting together the collective gift—these are all examples of elements that can be easily moved if it's necessary to create time for exploring what has come up in the moment.

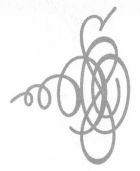
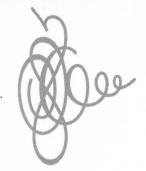

BE READY TO LET THE RITUAL MANIFEST AS IT NEEDS TO
HAPPEN . . . THIS ABILITY TO FLOW AND AD-LIB IS ANOTHER
SKILL THAT TAKES EXPERIENCE, BUT THAT HAPPENS IN TIME.

—Diane Stein, *Casting the Circle*

Trusting the Process

Every blessingway ritual has a tendency to take on a life or energy of its own! Even the most well-planned rituals cannot take into account what will happen synergistically when a group of women gather together. As a conduit for Spirit, trust that whatever is happening is happening for a reason. Keep this in mind, and you'll find that you can effectively guide the group—which includes evaluating whether various occurrences support or detract from the work of the blessingway. You can always decide to skip certain scheduled elements if the work has already been accomplished, albeit in an unintended way.

Even if you've got this concept, you may still secretly hope that the blessingway ritual will unfold in the way you've envisioned it. And though this may happen upon occasion, the reality is that it's unusual. There will be times when a ritual element is inadvertently left out. There will be times when you'll think that a particular piece was not "well done." There

will be times when you'll find yourself preoccupied with tallying up all the "mistakes" that you feel have been made. In these instances, the crucial thing to remember is this: even the most awkward or erroneous events that take place during a ritual are usually blessings in disguise. Everything always works out for the best, and in the end, you'll see that what you've gained from the experience is really of much greater value than what you felt you'd lost in the moment.

As you continue to lead more blessingways, you will find that you're paying more attention to the "passage" element of the ritual, as opposed to the "performance" element of the ritual. You will instinctively know how to leave space for things to happen, as opposed to trying to cover all the bases, and you will understand that oftentimes there is far more to be gained by letting go of the plan than by sticking to it. You will be able to trust, to surrender, and to allow a blessingway—similar to a birth—to simply unfold.

CHAPTER 10

Afterthoughts

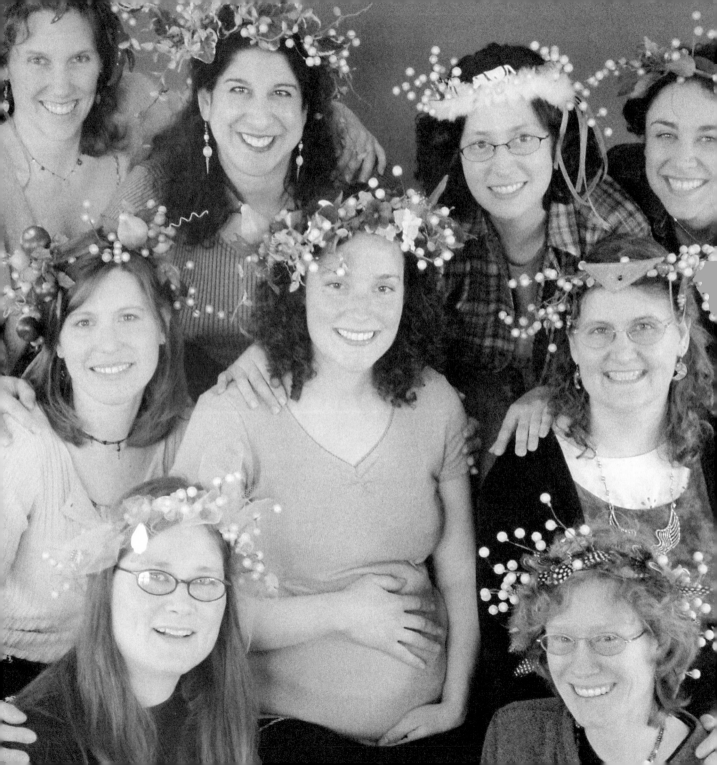

The Hopi **Tápu'at**, or **Mother and Child**, symbolizes the path to emergence and spiritual rebirth.

BLESSINGWAY RITUALS are incredibly powerful! Even after we think all has been said and done, after the last dish has been wiped dry, the last candle snuffed, the last piece of furniture pushed back into place with care and precision, we are left with a feeling of "wow." One last visual scan confirms that the ritual space is back in order. Even so, we find ourselves wandering around—checking and rechecking—for it often feels like it isn't all put away. We worry that something will be left behind. It took us a while to realize that, in fact, something is always left behind after a blessingway. We can't see it, but we can all feel it. An energy lingers. Something has changed. We have changed.

The amazing energies at work during a blessingway ritual are both powerful and transformative. By the end of the ritual, the mother-to-be is in a state of readiness for birthing and mothering, which the blessingway circle's initiatory nature has helped her attain. Many women with whom we've worked have sent us cards and letters that convey their thoughts, feelings, and heart's truth about their blessingway experience. Sometimes in their own words, sometimes borrowing the words of others, the profound effects of this life-changing ritual have been expressed quite beautifully:

- "After my blessingway, I felt beautiful for the first time since I could remember. Did I ever feel that way before? I honestly do not know."
- "I felt powerful and ready to deliver my baby. I know without a doubt that my blessingway helped me achieve my VBAC [Vaginal Birth after Cesarean]."
- "The red yarn wrapped around my wrist reminds me of the connection I have to women, that I am no less a woman because I'm birthing a baby from my heart instead of my physical body."
- "My blessingway was an amazing, transformative, and loving experience. It has truly provided me with strength in my darkest times, and it has been a personal source of pride and joy to have been welcomed into the ranks of mothers."
- "Thank you for holding me in your arms . . . it helps me know what my children know when I hold them."

Liminal Limbo

The span of time from the blessingway to birth and the postpartum stage is a critical period during which the mother-to-be/new mother will need the circle's continued support. When a woman leaves her blessingway, she may find that the world is not quite the same as before her ritual. She may feel that she has stepped into liminal space—a place between two very

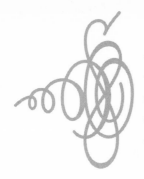

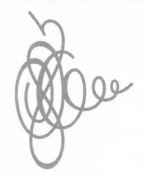

GIVING BIRTH IS PRIESTESS WORK; IT REQUIRES A WOMAN
TO PASS THROUGH A PAINFUL AND DANGEROUS INITIATION
IN WHICH SHE JOURNEYS TO THE THRESHOLD BETWEEN
WORLDS AND RISKS HER OWN LIFE TO HELP ANOTHER SOUL
CROSS OVER. —Jalaja Bonheim, *Aphrodite's Daughters*

different ways of life: an old way of life that she released during her ritual, and a new way of life that has not yet quite begun. During this liminal or threshold period, the mother-to-be may easily slip out of her altered state of readiness and into an uncertain state of limbo—a state in which the resources gathered during her blessingway can fall beyond her reach.

The length of this liminal period varies with each woman. (For instance, if the mother-to-be is adopting a child, her wait may be a long one.) In any case, it's very important that the mother-to-be keep her connection with her blessingway work strong during this waiting period, for she must remain poised for the work yet to come—that of taking her final steps into motherhood.

So how can we, her closest friends, support her in maintaining access to her achieved altered state, her feeling of readiness and empowerment? There are many ways to help the mother-to-be keep these gifts alive and in her conscious life until she needs to use them in her birthing and mothering. As part of her vital support team we can do any of the following:

- Create a blessingway altar for her in her home and encourage her to visit the altar daily.

- Send her prayers, energy, and blessings each time we notice our yarn bracelets from weaving the web.

- Remind her that when she sees her yarn bracelet, gift bead jewelry, or any other gifts or items from her blessingway, she can open her heart and reconnect to the energy that was raised, her web of women supporters, or any other empowering aspects of her ritual.

- Spend time with her meditatively, remembering and reexperiencing parts of her blessingway.

- Set a date with her (fairly soon after the blessingway) to help put together a blessingway scrapbook, string her gift beads, cast her belly, or do other reconnective activities.

- Suggest ways she might use this time for herself, such as reading fluffy fiction, having lunch with friends, seeing movies, or finishing projects.

- Encourage her to try "nesting"—sorting and reorganizing things at home; many women find it very comforting during this time.

- Make her a CD of the meditation and/or the music that was included during her blessingway.

- Remind her of how important it is to allow herself some self-indulgent activities, or pampering things to help her relax. Suggest massages, prenatal (and later, postpartum) yoga classes, or warm baths with scented oils and her blessingway music or any other music she loves.

- Suggest that she wear her hair down, or "unknotted," to symbolically facilitate the child's coming.

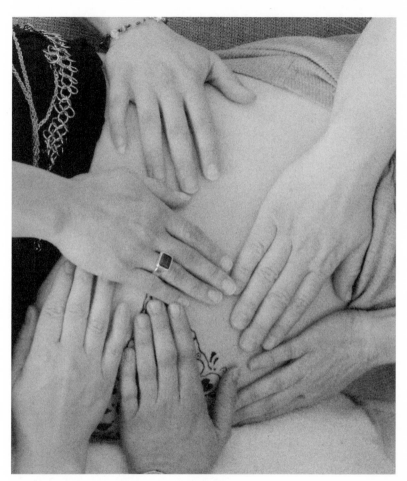

• Encourage her to think of her due date as a "due month," and let her know that the coming of labor may fall anywhere from two weeks before the estimated due date to two weeks after it. This may help free her to let things flow in their own natural course, within safe boundaries.

A LAYING-ON-OF-HANDS RITUAL

If the mother-to-be experiences ongoing anxiety, arrange for several women from the blessingway circle to set a date to go to her home and perform a laying-on-of-hands ritual. This will help her to get in touch with her baby and bring to light any concerns, expectations, or fears that need to be put to rest.

Two mothers we know felt their babies would never come when they were twelve and thirteen days past due date. In both cases, their blessingway circles went over to their homes to hold a laying-on-of-hands ritual. Insights were gained, and both moms went into labor within a day.

• Offer her affirmations, such as "I release my attachment to my baby's due date," if she is experiencing distracting thoughts, disquieting feelings, or growing worries. (This is a simple—but effective—way to help her release any discordant energies that are building within her.)

During a laying-on-of-hands ritual, we physically connect with the mother-to-be by placing our hands on her body in ways that feel comfortable to her. We then meditatively connect with the baby and wait to

111

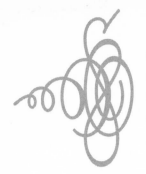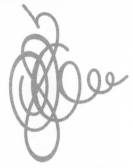

SUBCONSCIOUSLY, WE [MAY] KEEP THE BABY INSIDE, AFRAID OF
LETTING GO BECAUSE THE MINUTE WE LET GO TO ALLOW A NEW
LIFE TO ENTER THE WORLD, OUR NEW LIVES WILL BEGIN TOO.

—Carroll Dunham, *Mamatoto: A Celebration of Birth*

receive insights or messages. Here are the steps in the process:

- Select some soothing, long-playing meditation music and play it at a low level.

- Help the mother-to-be into a comfortable position on the floor (lying on her left side), and support her head, belly, and legs with soft pillows.

- Invite the women who are present for the ritual to sit closely around the mother-to-be. Make sure that they are comfortable enough to maintain extended physical contact with the mother-to-be, and that they touch the mother-to-be in a way that is comfortable for her as well.

- Select a leader to guide the group into a meditative state.

- The leader then invites everyone to close their eyes and to place their hands lovingly on the mother-to-be. She then begins the music and takes the women through a guided meditation (see the Laying-on-of-Hands Meditation sidebar).

- Let the circle do its work with the baby for as long as necessary. Invite the women to share any impressions or messages they receive with the mother-to-be as they arise. Encourage the mom to speak to anything that triggers a thought or emotion, and offer her supportive language for gaining clarity or releasing issues brought to light. You may spend from twenty minutes to an hour or

more doing this. (Just check in with the mom-to-be to make sure that she remains physically comfortable.)

- Ask for any last impressions, and then guide the ritual to a close. Be sure to help the mother-to-be up and into a comfortable position when it seems appropriate.

- Make plans for another visit and for ongoing support until the baby arrives, and remind everyone to keep their phone trees with them wherever they go!

Postpartum Support

As a culture, we are fairly good at paying attention to a mother-to-be throughout her pregnancy, labor, and delivery. However, we seem to have lost touch with how important it is to support a woman after her baby is born.

Hospitals, driven by insurance companies, have shortened postpartum stays without providing supplementary home care. Books and childbirth classes offer much valuable information, but they generally do not educate a woman adequately for what lies ahead: the long road of motherhood. Consequently, many of us find ourselves ill prepared for the issues that we face after our babies have been born.

It was once common for a woman's mother to

come and stay with her after she gave birth. These days, this does not happen often for a variety of reasons. Families are more spread out, our parents are continuing to work longer than they may have in the past, and many of us are choosing to have children later in life—which means that our parents are older, too. Whatever the reason—be it availability, capability, or in some cases, parent-daughter conflict—it is no longer a given that a woman will receive nurturing, support, or help from her family.

A blessingway connects the circle of women, creating a community. There is much we can do as members of this community to support to the new mother during the challenging postpartum period. We can:

- Nurture her and her family
- Provide her with emotional support and encouragement
- Be a safe person with whom she can talk about the birth
- Support her throughout hormonal ups and downs
- Help facilitate her physical healing process
- Make and bring over healing ointments or teas (see the

Laying-on-of-Hands Meditation

Take one long, deep breath in. Hold that for a moment, then slowly blow it out. Now allow your breath to flow in and out at its own pace, naturally, gently, and quietly. Become aware of your body. Notice any tight spots. Now imagine that you can send your breath to that spot, as if your in-breath could stretch and relax that area, and your out-breath could release any remaining tension and carry it away. Repeat this process on your own for the next few moments. (Pause.) Now take one more deep breath in to stretch and relax your body as a whole, then release that breath to let go of anything you don't need.

Bring all your attention gently toward (name of the mother-to-be)'s baby. See or sense the baby, warm and secure in its womb home, and extend a quiet greeting. Offer the baby words of encouragement, safety, and peace. When you feel complete with that, gently ask the baby whether there are any concerns or fears to be cleared out of the way in order to come out and meet us, and listen openheartedly with all your senses. Everyone receives information differently—some through words, others through pictures, sounds, or physical sensations. Simply accept what comes, and when you feel ready, share what you've been given with the mother-to-be and the circle, allowing a meditative dialogue to follow. (Gather and share impressions for as long as necessary.)

(Name of the mother-to-be), send your baby your love and affection. Tell your baby how much you look forward to being able to hold him or her in your arms and say, "See you soon!" Now, let's all bid the baby good-bye until next we meet, gently withdrawing our attention, leaving behind our love and caring like a warm and peaceful cradle. Turn your attention to your own body as you gently withdraw your hand from (name of the mother-to-be). Take a slow, deep breath in, then slowly breathe out; become more fully aware of your body seated here. When you feel fully present to yourself, slowly open your eyes to let them gradually adjust to the light in the room.

Lavender Moon's Postpartum Healing Compress sidebar.)

- Assist her with breastfeeding
- Hold her baby (so she may nap or take a shower)
- Run errands, prepare meals, and help out with household tasks
- Provide care for her other children and her pets
- Answer questions about basic infant care
- Offer parenting tips and provide resources
- Share our own personal experiences

The support we have to offer a new mother will not only be invaluable, it may also help minimize feelings of being overwhelmed and the frustration that so often occurs during the postpartum period. Simply reminding and reassuring her that, in just a few short weeks, everything will become familiar, even routine, may help her gain confidence as a new mom.

It is not easy for most of us to ask for help, even when we desperately need it. So it's important that we don't wait for a new mom to call upon us, because that may not happen. By wearing our yarn bracelets until a new mom feels settled into her new role, we are reminded not only to keep her in our thoughts and prayers, but to extend ourselves to her by making specific offers and asking questions such as:

- "How are your meals going?"
- "What can I pick up for you at the store?"
- "How about if I run some laundry for you?"
- "Let me wash those dishes."

- "Have you had anything to eat lately?"
- "Are you drinking lots of water?"

When we encourage a new mother to accept the help she really does need with the everyday work of running a household, we help her honor this sacred postpartum time by freeing her to rest, heal, and bond with her new baby. Our collective gifts of service will enable her to practice the self-nurturing that is often hard to do (for example, perhaps she can sleep when the baby sleeps, instead of rushing around to get chores done). It's important that we remember to be mindful, however, when visiting a new mom or offering our assistance that we not add stress to her already complicated life.

Sometimes a new mother's needs extend beyond our availability or experience. When this occurs, we may best help by referring her to outside resources, such as La Leche League, a postpartum doula, a midwife, a counselor, or a physician.

HIRING A POSTPARTUM DOULA

If a new mother's friends or family are unable to meet her support needs for any reason, it may be wise to suggest that she hire a postpartum doula. *Doula,* the Greek word for servant, has come to mean a woman who serves or "mothers" a new mother.

A doula can provide a family with invaluable support before, during, and after the birth of their child. A postpartum doula can help a new mom (and dad) move into parenthood with more ease by providing both emotional and physical support. (See page 139 for more information.)

Lavender Moon's Postpartum Healing Compress

This easy-to-make and very effective herbal compress can be used to heal and soothe a new mother's perineum after her baby's birth or to treat engorged breasts.

3 tablespoons finely chopped fresh ginger root

2 tablespoons dried comfrey root or leaf

2 tablespoons dried plantain leaf

2 tablespoons dried yarrow

2 tablespoons dried Saint-John's-wort flowers

8 to 12 cups water

Simmer fresh ginger root in water in a saucepan for ½ hour. Add herbs, and then steep on low for another 10 minutes. Strain into a large bowl. (Note: This herbal tea can be reused and reheated for up to two days.)

For perineum: Immerse a small clean towel in the hot tea, wring, then apply to the new mother's perineum. When the cloth cools, repeat the process. Continue the application for up to 20 minutes. Use it several times a day during the first week following birth.

The steeped herbal mixture may also be strained directly into a sitz bath or into a perineal rinse bottle to be squeezed over the perineal area when using the bathroom.

For engorged breasts: Immerse a small clean towel in the hot tea, wring, then wrap it completely around the new mother's breast and under her armpit.

CONTACTING LA LECHE LEAGUE

La Leche League is a volunteer-based international organization whose goal is to give information and encouragement to all women who wish to breastfeed. Facilitated La Leche League groups meet monthly to discuss the various issues that women face during birth, postpartum, and while parenting their children. The meetings follow a four-topic cycle: (1) the advantages of breastfeeding, (2) the family and the breastfed baby during early post-partum, (3) breastfeeding techniques and problem solving, and (4) nutrition for the lactating mother and her children.

La Leche League leaders have firsthand experience as moms themselves. They volunteer their time enthusiastically, and they are happy to offer support or guidance by phone at any time of day or night. If the need arises, some leaders will even provide postpartum home visits to assist or advise a new mother who is breastfeeding. (See page 139 for more information.)

Sharing This Knowledge

The information contained within *Mother Rising* came to us in waves. The first wave came from books, pamphlets, and newsletters written by women who had already begun to explore rituals and blessingways. Excited by what we read, we consciously began to incorporate the concepts we were uncovering into the ritual work we were doing.

The next wave came through our actual experiences: the more rituals we created, the more we knew about ritual. As we neared the end of this book project, we realized that a great deal of knowledge was coming to us intuitively and that we seemed to have gained access to some mysterious pool of information. We now recognize that this "mysterious pool" is actually the collective feminine spirit.

Every woman who does this important work contributes her discoveries to that very same pool, and in turn, that information is made available to women everywhere. By heightening our awareness and creating conscious connections with one another, we will all gain the ability to tap into our collective feminine spirit, and thereby gain access to all the knowledge and wisdom of women who have walked the path before us.

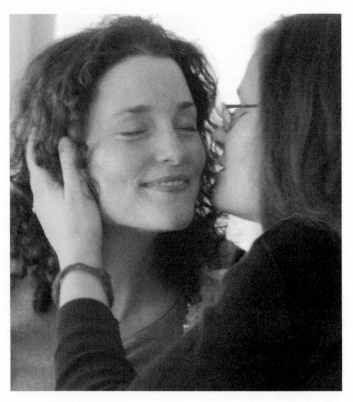

Tools and Resources

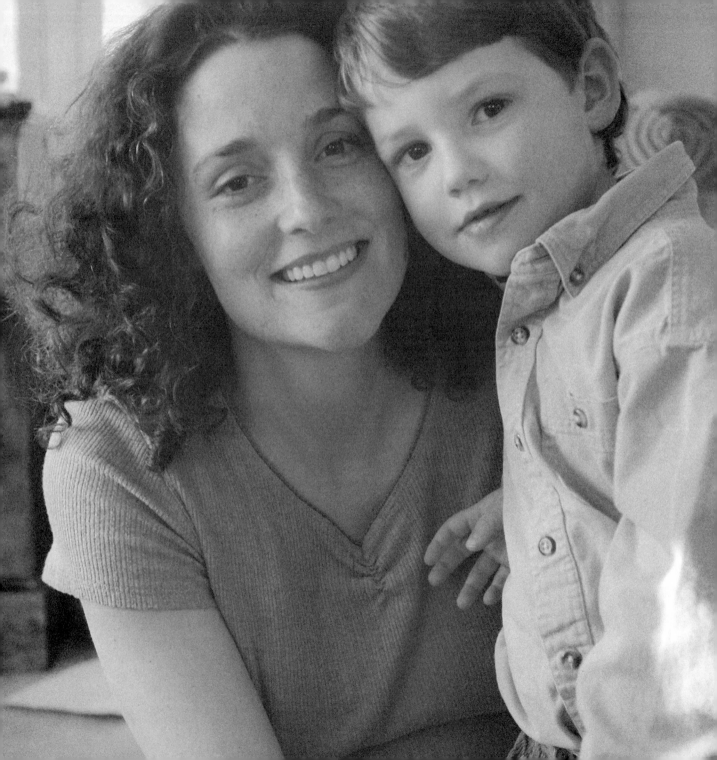

Blessingway Planning Checklist

THREE MONTHS BEFORE THE BABY'S DUE DATE

Review chapter 2, "Planning a Blessingway" (page 13). Then do the following:

- Form your planning team
- Meet with the mother-to-be
- Set the blessingway date
- Create the guest list
- Choose the location
- Send out save the date cards or emails
- Assign roles and responsibilities

Next review chapter 3, "Designing Your Ritual" (page 23) and chapters 4 through 8, which present the five stages of a ritual. Then flesh out your plans as follows:

- Create your ritual outline
- Create a ritual supplies list

ONE MONTH BEFORE THE BLESSINGWAY

Meet with your planning team to finalize the event details. Now is also the time to make the following arrangements:

- Create and send out invitations
- Visit the blessingway location to assess ritual space, amenities, parking, and so on

ONE WEEK BEFORE THE BLESSINGWAY

Review chapter 9, "Leading a Blessingway" (page 97). It's time to fine-tune your plans:

- Finalize the ritual outline
- Schedule a rehearsal

ONE DAY BEFORE THE BLESSINGWAY

Get everything ready:

- Begin preparing the ritual site (provide housecleaning, if necessary)
- Confirm event arrival time with all organizers and leaders
- Pack all supplies

THE DAY OF THE BLESSINGWAY

Two to three hours before the guests arrive, set the stage:

- Arrange furniture, create altars, set up ritual supplies, arrange flowers, get familiar with the music system, mix the henna (if using any), set up for the feast, set out snacks and drinks
- Review the ritual outline and supplies list. Make sure that you have everything you need for your ritual (think carefully—you don't want to find yourself scrambling around to locate something during the ritual).

One hour before the guests arrive, prepare the ritual space and leaders:

- Clear the atmosphere and reset the energy (if desired at this time)
- Prepare yourself and the other leaders
- Check in with everyone, then perform the centering ritual

As the guests arrive, welcome them:

- Start playing music that will set the special tone for the day
- Greet everyone and tell them what to do with their things
- Confirm heating or refrigeration instructions for feast dishes
- Relax, breathe, and have a wonderful blessingway!

After the ritual, take care of follow-up details:

- Assign someone to finish making any gifts that still need to be constructed (such as jewelry, a quilt, or a mobile). Don't make the mom-to-be wait too long—plan to complete and return her gifts to her as soon as possible!
- Verify that all guests have received a copy of the phone tree, labor candles, and anything else to be shared
- Check in with the mom-to-be about a tentative postpartum meal schedule, or put out a sign-up sheet (see the Coordinating Post-Blessingway Meals sidebar, page 21)
- Ask for volunteers to stay and help clean up

AFTER THE BLESSINGWAY EVENT

Review chapter 10, "Afterthoughts" (page 107). Continue to keep the circle's energy focused on the mother-to-be while she still needs it:

- Check in with the mom-to-be regularly to assess her energy and her needs
- Work with the women from the blessingway circle to ensure that the mom-to-be receives the support she requires
- Follow up with the person(s) assigned to finish constructing any collective gift. Has the gift been completed? Has the mother-to-be received it?
- Follow up with the gifts of service coordinator to ensure that a schedule has been created, and that the meals or other services are, in fact, being delivered

Blessingway Supplies Checklist

The following sections include items that are commonly used in rituals and supplies that pertain to specific blessingway elements.

GENERAL RITUAL SUPPLIES

You will probably need most of the following items for your blessingway ritual:

- Books containing readings or prayers
- CD or cassette player (or access to music equipment)
- Cushions, chairs, or BackJack portable chairs
- Matches
- Music CDs or cassettes
- Musical instruments
- Pitcher of water and cups
- Scissors
- Small clock or wristwatch
- Snack mix (see recipe, page 88)
- Tissues (for cleanup, weeping, or runny noses)
- Water (if there is no access to water)

SPECIFIC ACTIVITY SUPPLIES

You can select items from whichever of the following ritual elements you will be including in your blessingway:

BUILDING AN ALTAR

- Candles
- Compass (for determining each direction's location)
- Fresh flowers
- Symbolic items
- Tablecloths
- Tables

CASTING A BELLY

- Instructions (see page 60)
- Pan (shallow)
- Paper towels
- Petroleum jelly (or alternative)
- Plaster bandages
- Plastic or tarps (large)
- Scissors

OR

- Art materials
- Finished belly cast

CLEARING THE SPACE OR HOUSE

- Bells, rattles, or other musical instruments
- Smudging supplies
- Water purification supplies

FEASTING

- Centerpiece or vase of flowers
- Coffeemaker, coffee, cream/creamer, and sugar
- Coolers
- Garbage bags (large, for cleanup)
- Ice
- Music CDs or cassettes
- Tablecloth
- Tableware
- Teapot and assorted teas
- Trivets and hotpads

GIVING GIFTS

- Bowls or baskets (to hold gift beads and other symbolic objects)
- Paper and pen (for the scribe to record gifts)
- Supplies for creating a collective gift

MAKING A WREATH

- Flowers and herbs, fresh or dried
- Ribbons
- Wire
- Wreath form
- Hot glue gun and glue sticks

MAKING JEWELRY

- Instructions (see page 70)
- Gift beads
- Filler beads
- Crimp beads
- Jewelry wire
- Needle-nose pliers
- Scissors
- Split rings
- Spring ring or lobster clasp

PAMPERING

- Crown or special clothing
- Fresh or dried herbs for footbath (for recipe see page 63)
- Hairbrush (mother-to-be should bring her own)
- Hair clips, ribbons, fasteners, and/or beads
- Massage oil or lotion
- Mehndi kit or supplies (see Recommended Resources for sources)
- Scented bath oils
- Soap

- Towels
- Tub (for soaking feet)

- Bowl (for incense cones or dried herbs, or for tamping out a smudge stick)
- Feather (for fanning the smoke)
- Matches
- Smudge stick, dried herbs, or incense
- Tin foil (to cover the bowl, or to wrap the smudge stick in when done)

- Bowl
- Fresh rose petals or rose oil
- Hand towel
- Sea salt (about 1 tablespoon per quart of water)
- Water

- Alcohol
- Dried herbs (for recipe see page 55)
- Epsom salts
- Fireproof bowl (big enough to hold a tuna can)
- Matches
- Trivet or hot pad
- Tuna can
OR
- Covered container
- Paper and pens

- Matches
- Paper and pens
- Symbolic (or other) items to be burned
- Wood and kindling

- Ball of yarn
- Scissors

Feminine Expressions of the Divine

The Goddess can be worked with as a concept or in a specific form. (See Recommended Resources to learn more.) The following is a sampling of some of her many faces.

- Moon goddess of love, fertility, and protection
- Blesses us with fertility and protection
- Good to summon for protecting a mother and conceiving a child

- Is there a strong female ancestor in the mother-to-be's family? Perhaps calling upon the relative's memory will assist her in building her confidence during her blessingway for giving birth
- Blesses us with her personal strengths and gifts
- Good to summon for situations where her qualities would be helpful

ARTEMIS (GREEK)

- Virgin goddess of the moon and protectoress of childbirth and women; thought to be the equivalent of the Roman goddess Diana
- Blesses us with courage and independence
- Good to summon for self-discipline and developing physical strength

ARTEMIS OF EPHESUS (AMAZONIAN)

- Multi-breasted Mother goddess
- Blesses us with fertility and protection
- Good to summon for protecting mother and child during childbirth

BASTET (EGYPTIAN)

- Goddess of love and fertility
- Blesses us with nurturance and fertility
- Good to summon for nurturing capabilities for mothering

BRIGIT (CELTIC)

- Goddess of healing, prophecy, and inspiration; fire deity and patron of the hearth
- Blesses us with a perfect balance of femininity and "no apologies" power
- Good to summon for courage and protection

CERES (ROMAN)

- Goddess of bountiful harvest and growth; thought to be the equivalent of the Greek goddess Demeter
- Blesses us with fertility and a safe and successful pregnancy

- Good to summon for conceiving a child, protection, and ensuring a healthy baby

CHANGING WOMAN (NATIVE AMERICAN)

- A Great Mother who represents the cycle of life and all the seasons
- Blesses us with grounding and growth through change
- Good to summon for opening to mothering instincts and connecting to nature

DAMARA (BRITISH)

- Goddess of home and hearth who helps with family harmony
- Blesses us with peaceful energy within the domestic realm and abundance
- Good to summon for peace in the home, and guiding and healing children

DANA (CELTIC)

- Creator goddess, Great Mother aspect of the Creator
- Blesses us with fertility and the ability to nurture
- Good to summon for conceiving a child and acquiring strong mothering qualities

DEMETER (GREEK)

- Goddess of the Earth, Mother goddess; thought to be the equivalent of the Roman goddess Ceres
- Blesses us with the ability to nurture, care take, love, and heal
- Good to summon for nursing relationships, mother-daughter bond with female children, or nurturing yourself or others

DEVI (HINDU)

- Vedic goddess, known as the Universal Mother or Great Mother
- Blesses us with the feminine spirit and a connection to the Divine
- Good to summon for divine guidance, birthing, and mothering support

DIANA (ROMAN)

- Virgin goddess of hunting and the moon; thought to be the equivalent of the Greek goddess Artemis
- Blesses us with strength, purification, power, and protection
- Good to summon for a painless childbirth

THE DIVINE MOTHER

- A general name for the concept of divine motherly guidance
- Blesses us with strength, support, and motherly knowing
- Good to summon for accessing the ability, strength, and courage to mother

GABRIEL (ARCHANGEL)

- This well-known angel (interpreted sometimes as female, sometimes as male) told Elizabeth and Mary of the impending births of their sons, John the Baptist and Jesus of Nazareth
- Blesses us with strength and courage
- Good to summon for conception, watching over the adoption of a child, and help with delivering messages to and from the Divine

THE GODDESS

- A general archetype expressing the spirit of the feminine divine
- Blesses us with intuition and fertility
- Good to summon for divine guidance, protection, and conception

HATHOR (EGYPTIAN)

- Goddess of the sun, sky, newborns, and the dead
- Blesses us with love and fertility
- Good to summon for conception, protecting pregnant women (acts as a midwife) and newborns, help with raising children

HERA (GREEK)

- Goddess of marriage and personal power; Sky Queen; triple goddess representing youth, prime, and age; thought to be the equivalent of the Roman goddess Juno
- Blesses us with wisdom and insight into feminine issues
- Good to summon for guiding women through life passages and assistance with mothering

HESTIA (GREEK)

- Goddess of hearth and home; goddess of the public hearth as well, she embodied the spirit of community; thought to be the equivalent of the Roman goddess Vesta
- Blesses us with family unity and community spirit
- Summon for guiding and protecting the family and home, help with extended family and community issues

ISHTAR (MESOPOTAMIAN)
• Goddess of sexual love and fertility
• Blesses us with compassion, healing, and gentleness
• Summon for conception and parenting assistance

ISIS (EGYPTIAN)
• Moon goddess who embodies total femininity and motherhood, noted for her great love of her husband and child; mother of the Sun God Horus, she was a great teacher of womanly arts, a culture-bringer, and healer; so powerful that she could even overcome fate
• Blesses us with the ability to love and nurture
• Good to summon for manifesting Divine Mother energy

IX CHEL (MAYAN)
• The Queen, the Mother, Our Mother, the White Lady, and the Goddess of Becoming; a goddess of fertility, childbirth, water, weaving, the moon, and medicine; a protector of children
• Blesses us with the safety of our young, and the mystery and joy of our female sexuality
• Good to summon for protection during childbirth, protecting children in general

JUNO (ROMAN:
• Goddess of women, time, and the menstrual cycle, she had many names relating to the various stages of women's reproductive lives; leads us through life passages, and is a giver of warnings; thought to be the equivalent of the Greek goddess Hera
• Blesses us with women's wisdom, protection, and guidance

• Good to summon for showing us the way to motherhood and ensuring our safety

KUAN YIN, ALSO KWAN YIN OR QUAN YIN (CHINESE)
• Goddess of compassion and protection (especially for women and children)
• Blesses us with compassion, feminine grace, beauty, power, kindness, gentleness, and sweetness toward self and others
• Good to summon for protecting women and children

LILITH (SUMERIAN/HEBREW)
• The first female according to Genesis; goddess of equality for women; chose her own path (rather than subordination to Adam), and consequently left the Garden of Eden
• Blesses us with self-awareness, personal power, and freedom of choice
• Good to summon for support in new life choices and revealing deep inner truths

LUCINA (SWEDISH/ROMAN, AS ANOTHER FORM OF JUNO)
• Goddess of light, she is the first light seen after birth; a goddess of labor and the childbed
• Blesses us with the ability to untangle problems and shed light on dark issues
• Good to summon for easing labor pain and making sure all goes well in childbirth

MAMI (SUMERIAN)
• Mother Goddess; midwife of the gods; created the earth and all its beings

- Blesses us with nurturing and creativity
- Good to summon for power for birthing and protection during childbirth

MOTHER EARTH, ALSO GAIA OR EA
- The spiritual nature of the earth itself
- Blesses us with grounding and protection
- Good to summon for drawing strength from the earth, and staying conscious of the earthly work of birthing while accessing spiritual wisdom and power

NUT (EGYPTIAN)
- Goddess of the Sky; mother of Isis; very protective Mother goddess; often depicted with a water pot on her head, which is thought to represent the womb (her name is correctly pronounced Nu-it)
- Blesses us with protection and a safe container for difficult work
- Good to summon for protection during childbirth, and casting a strong, safe, supportive circle for blessingways

SHE WHO HEALS (NATIVE AMERICAN)
- Midwife, herbalist, medicine woman, spirit healer, and teacher of the cycles of the earth walk; she is the keeper of the healing arts, mother of all rites of passage, and guardian of the mysteries of life and death
- Blesses us with healing, wisdom, and guidance
- Good to summon for guidance during childbirth, spiritual wisdom, and safe passage

VENUS OF WILLENDORF (ANCIENT MOTHER)
- Paleolithic Mother goddess; statue (found near what is now Willendorf, Austria) dates back to 25,000 to 20,000 BCE, and is the earliest known representation of a woman
- Blesses us with natural femaleness, fertility, power, and beauty
- Good to summon for conception and help with nurturing children from one stage of life to another

VESTA (ROMAN)
- Goddess of hearth, home, and strength (rekindled through the continued renewal of the family); thought to be the equivalent of the Greek goddess Hestia
- Blesses us with family unity and power—renewed and restored through the family's strength and regeneration
- Good to summon for guidance and protecting the family and home

VIRGIN MARY (MOTHER OF CHRIST)
- The Queen of Heaven and the angels; gave birth to God on earth as Jesus through a virgin conception
- Blesses us with fertility, healing, patience, kindness, and the ability to be loving
- Good to summon for adopting children and help with any issue related to children (especially helpful to those working with children)

YEMAYA (AFRICAN)
- Associated with the moon, the ocean, and female mysteries; governs the household; intervenes in

women's affairs; invoked by women for aid in childbirth, love, and healing; watches over the conception and birth of children and ensures their safety during childhood

- Blesses us with compassion, wisdom, inspiration, and female power
- Good to summon for healing, comfort, making whole that which is incomplete, acquiring ancient wisdom, protecting the home, help with learning not to give your power away, comforting children in crisis, and washing away sorrow

Symbolism

The use of symbolic objects and imagery will deepen and support your ritual experience.

ANIMAL SYMBOLISM

Animals represent certain qualities, and their presence can help your ritual work:

- **Ant:** patience, hard work
- **Antelope:** action, grace
- **Bear:** introspection, hibernation, deliberateness, earthly power
- **Beaver:** building, planning, industriousness, energy, bravery
- **Bee:** productivity, happiness when busy
- **Beetle (scarab):** rebirth, resurrection
- **Blue bird:** happiness, freedom
- **Buffalo:** abundance, wealth
- **Bull:** tenacity, strength, groundedness
- **Butterfly:** transformation, lightheartedness, joy
- **Cat:** nurturing, clarity of sight, dexterity, cleverness, independence

- **Crane:** joy, loyalty, good luck, prosperity, purity, vitality, long life
- **Crow:** sacred law, change
- **Deer:** peace, gentleness, kindness, lovingness
- **Dog:** loyalty, persistence, a good friend
- **Dolphin:** breath, inspiration
- **Dragonfly:** illusions revealed, wisdom, enlightenment, transformation
- **Eagle:** Spirit, honesty, divine connection, the balance of Spirit grounded in our everyday lives
- **Elephant:** ancient memory, regal presence
- **Frog:** cleansing, excitement
- **Giraffe:** big picture, large heart
- **Grouse:** sacred spiral of birth and rebirth
- **Hawk:** messages, broad view, hunter, clarity
- **Hippo:** mothering, protective presence at births
- **Horse:** power—both physical and otherworldly, vision, courage, intuition
- **Hummingbird:** joy, love, openheartedness, pure bliss of life
- **Lamb:** innocence, new beginnings, self-sacrifice, joyful abandon
- **Lioness:** assertion of the feminine, protection of the family, courage
- **Otter:** balanced female energy—playful and powerful
- **Owl:** wisdom, cutting clarity, awareness of deception, appreciation of the beauty of the dark
- **Panther:** one's true power
- **Porcupine:** innocence, protection
- **Prairie dog:** community, playfulness
- **Rabbit:** fertility, abundant new life, quickness, intelligence, caution, fearfulness

- **Raven:** transmutation, magic, mystical change
- **Rhino:** self-confidence, impatience
- **Seal:** imagination, women's work, balanced emotions
- **Snake:** passion, renewal of self, transmutation
- **Spider:** creation, connections, creativity
- **Squirrel:** gathering, planning ahead
- **Swan:** grace, evolution, potential
- **Tiger:** passion, the beauty of power
- **Turkey:** giving, transcending self, sacredness of life
- **Turtle:** Mother Earth, patience, deliberateness, wisdom, peace
- **Whale:** vastness, divine wisdom, ability to navigate the sea of emotions
- **White buffalo:** answered prayers
- **Wolf:** teacher, guardian of the family

COLOR SYMBOLISM

Colors, which can help guide a ritual's energy, have many associations:

- **Black** is protection, rest, birth, shadows, mysteries of the subconscious mind, magic, and banishing. It absorbs negativity, and perhaps that is why Western mourners wear black. Black is the color of the West (Native American tradition).
- **Blue** is communication, truth, tranquility, happiness, and water. The blue sea is the subconscious mind, the feminine, the Great Mother, and deep secrets. The blue sky is the conscious mind, the masculine, and the Great Father. Blue is the color of the West (Wiccan tradition).
- **Green** is love, healing, prosperity, fertility, new growth, and balance. It brings harmony, peace, reassurance, and contentment. Green is the color of the North (Wiccan tradition).
- **Orange** is joyful, optimistic, confident, flamboyant, warmhearted and tolerant. It represents the harvest, and it brings a sense of community.
- **Purple** is spirituality, truth seeking, love, honor, intuition, ancient wisdom, psychic perception, mystery, and enchantment. It facilitates and strengthens our connection to the Divine.
- **Red** is love, passion, sex, fire, anger, and courage. It is the symbol of life and creation because it is the color of blood. Red is the color of the South (Native American and Wiccan traditions).
- **White** is purity, innocence, cleanliness, purification, truth, protection, spiritual advancement, and openness to the realm of the divine. It contains all colors. It is virgin, pristine, and unsullied. White is the color of the North (Native American tradition).
- **Yellow** is uplifting. It brings trust, attraction, communication, movement, and power. It is air, the intellect, and the color of the sun. Yellow is the color of the East (Native American and Wiccan traditions).

FLOWER AND PLANT SYMBOLISM

Flowers and plants lend many healing qualities to support a ritual:

- **Baby's breath:** fertility
- **Borage:** courage
- **Buttercup:** joy, youth, new directions, self-worth
- **Carnation:** pride, beauty
- **Chamomile:** centering, peace, protection, healing
- **Chrysanthemum:** longevity, ease, vigor

- **Clover:** luck, love, fidelity
- **Daisy:** life, awareness, creativity, the sun, love, innocence, fidelity, dawn, new beginnings
- **Dandelion:** divination, welcoming, messages, foresight, oracles
- **Day lily:** Chinese symbol for mother
- **Gardenia:** action, purpose, protection, well-being
- **Heather:** grounding, beauty, spiritual transformation
- **Hyacinth:** reliability, constancy
- **Iris:** inspiration, rebirth
- **Lavender:** sleep, long life, wishes, peace, protection
- **Lilac:** clarity, productivity, spiritual balance, love, youth, joy, fastidiousness
- **Lotus:** harmony, serenity, many layers or levels of self
- **Marigold:** cares, burdens, change, luck in love, prophecy, legal matters, psychic energy, seeing magical creatures
- **Mistletoe:** luck, protection, fertility, dreams
- **Morning glory:** new beginnings, spontaneity
- **Nasturtium:** balance
- **Pansy:** glee, fancy, fondness
- **Periwinkle:** protection, rebirth, healing
- **Rose:** love, friendship, luck, protection
- **Rosebud:** new life
- **Snapdragon:** guidance, strength, expression, protection
- **Tulip:** success, trust, discernment, grounding, declaration of love
- **Violet:** simplicity, peace, stillness, grace, modesty, excellence, expression

FOOD SYMBOLISM

Foods, including culinary herbs and spices, nourish souls as well as bodies during a ritual:

- **Anise:** protection, purification, awareness, joy
- **Apple:** health, vitality, earth magic, grounding, knowledge
- **Apricot:** romance
- **Artichoke:** growth, safety
- **Avocado:** beauty
- **Banana:** heroic energy, male sexuality
- **Barley:** love, controlling pain
- **Basil:** protection, love, wealth, healing relationships, courage, fertility, fidelity
- **Beans:** divination, prosperity, decision making
- **Beef:** grounding
- **Beets:** passion, love, beauty
- **Blueberry:** peace, calm
- **Bread:** earth, the body, unity of spirit, kinship, sustenance, life
- **Broccoli:** strength, leadership, physical improvements
- **Cake:** sweetness in life, prosperity, celebration, joyous occasions
- **Cardamom:** strong unions and partnerships
- **Carrot:** vision, masculine energy
- **Cauliflower:** lunar- and water-related magic
- **Celery:** passion, grounding, peace
- **Cheese:** joy, health, fruition
- **Cherry:** love, female sexuality
- **Chicken:** health, well-being
- **Chives:** protection, breaking bad habits
- **Chocolate:** lifting emotions, love, pleasure

129

- **Cinnamon:** spiritual quest, power, love, success, safety, healing, protection, happy home
- **Clove:** stolen kisses, fun, love, dispelling negativity, seeing through illusions, protection, money
- **Coconut:** diversity, flexibility, spirituality
- **Coffee:** energy, alertness, mental awareness
- **Cookies:** maternal instincts, nurturing love
- **Coriander:** protection of home, peace, longevity, love, security, well-being, intelligence
- **Corn:** life of the land, cycles, eternity, sustenance (one of the three sacred foods of the northeastern Native Americans—corn, beans, and squash)
- **Cornmeal:** luck, protection, prosperity
- **Cranberry:** security, protection
- **Date:** resurrection, eternity, spirit
- **Dill:** protecting children
- **Egg:** fertility, new life, birth, mysticism, ancient questions, the sacred, safe container for spiritual transformation (the alchemical egg)
- **Fennel seed:** purification, protection, healing, prosperity
- **Fruit:** abundance, rewards, reaping harvest
- **Fruit, round:** fertility, nourishment
- **Garlic:** protection, healing, courage
- **Ginger:** vibrant energy, zeal, cleansing, health, power, success, love
- **Grains:** prosperity, potential for life, abundance, faith, sustenance
- **Grape:** dreams, visions, fertility
- **Grapefruit:** purification, the sun, health
- **Guava:** romance, fantasy, relieving sorrow
- **Hazelnut:** wisdom

- **Honey:** happiness, sweet things in life, the life force in all things (food of the gods)
- **Jelly:** joy, pleasantries
- **Juice:** rejuvenation, vitality
- **Lemon:** cleansing, purifying, love, marriage, blessings, joy, faithfulness
- **Lettuce:** financial magic, peace, relaxation
- **Lime:** cleansing
- **Melon:** wholeness, the brain, opportunity
- **Milk:** the Goddess, energy, maternal instinct, nurturing
- **Mint:** money, healing, strength, augmenting power
- **Mustard:** faith, mental alertness
- **Oats:** life of the land, prosperity, sustenance
- **Olive:** peace, spiritual pursuits
- **Onion:** layers, sadness
- **Orange:** the sun, happiness, health, love
- **Oyster:** hidden treasures, transforming irritations into gifts of great beauty
- **Parsley:** victory, desires, protection, luck, breaking old habits, protection from accidents
- **Pea:** the Goddess, magic, love
- **Peanut:** earth magic
- **Pear:** longevity, luck
- **Pepper, black:** cleansing, purification, protection, banishing
- **Pepper, green:** growth, prosperity
- **Pepper, red:** energy, vitality, strength
- **Pepper, white:** mystical transformation
- **Pepper, yellow:** empowered creativity
- **Pineapple:** healing, protection, prosperity, hospitality
- **Pomegranate:** fertility, the womb; the cycle of birth, death, and reincarnation

- **Popcorn:** lifting burdens
- **Pork:** fertility, profuseness
- **Potato:** health, grounding, earth magic
- **Quince:** happiness
- **Raspberry:** vigor, stamina, love
- **Rice:** fertility, abundant blessings
- **Rosemary:** bonding, healing, sleep, purification, cleansing, protection, clear thinking, youth, improving memory
- **Sage:** longevity, wishes, wisdom, fertility
- **Salmon:** moving ahead against all odds
- **Salt:** cleansing, purification, dispelling negativity, strength, stability
- **Strawberry:** zest, intensity, romance
- **Sweet potato:** well-foundedness, gentle love
- **Syrup:** tree magic, amiable meetings
- **Tea:** friendship, insight, relaxation
- **Thyme:** sleep, psychic energy, courage, healing
- **Tomato:** attracting love
- **Vegetables, green:** rebirth
- **Venison:** high energy, earth, sacred food
- **Wine:** spirit, blood, transcendence

GEM, STONE, AND SHELL SYMBOLISM

Gems, stones, and shells are beautiful objects that are infused with power and meaning:

- **Abalone:** brings forth inner wisdom, peace, tranquility, harmony, and emotional fluidity; is associated with feminine power and majesty
- **Agate:** brings strength and bravery, grounds, helps morning sickness, gives one the ability to discern the truth and accept circumstances
- **Agate, blue lace:** calms the mind, negates stubbornness, enhances psychic abilities
- **Agate, leopard skin:** attracts the opposite sex, aids with fertility, is associated with mystery
- **Agate, moss:** enhances connection to nature, aids growth, cleanses
- **Alexandrite:** brings joy and a sense of oneness with life
- **Amber:** heals, sooths, and harmonizes; activates altruistic nature; spiritualizes the intellect; protects health
- **Amethyst:** alleviates stress, raises hopes, brings purity and radiance, enhances connection to the divine and universal truths, aids in releasing negative thought patterns, has healing and calming properties, is very protective
- **Aquamarine:** brings peace, love, and purification; prevents miscarriage; has calming properties
- **Aventurine:** enhances visionary powers, intuition, and perception; brings good luck, prosperity, and emotional tranquility; supports independence, health, well-being, and a positive attitude toward life; aids in releasing anxiety and fear; brings one into alignment with their center
- **Bloodstone:** offers protection and inner guidance; prevents injury and stops bleeding; is a powerful physical healer; is associated with victory, wealth, and idealism
- **Carnelian:** enhances attunement with inner self; warms, brings joy, and opens the heart; stimulates conception, energy, passion, and creative expression; facilitates concentration and communication with higher self and spirit guides; is a highly evolved healer

- **Chalcedony:** aids with lactation; brings peace, protection (especially against nightmares), luck, and safe travel
- **Citrine:** enhances self-esteem and mental clarity, brings abundance and material well-being
- **Coral:** regulates menstruation; offers wisdom and protection
- **Diamond:** enhances spirituality, faithfulness, and reconciliation; offers protection and strength; heals sexual dysfunction
- **Emerald:** brings physical healing and protection, lends insight and security in love
- **Garnet:** protects and enhances bodily strength, invokes and releases one's inner fire
- **Gold:** enhances personal illumination and success; is associated with solar energy, the sun, and male aspects
- **Hematite:** grounds and heals, dissolves negative energy, decreases inflammation
- **Jade:** radiates divine, unconditional love; is associated with longevity, wisdom, protection, and prosperity
- **Jasper:** relieves pain and protects mother and child during childbirth, reduces fear, enhances health and beauty
- **Lapis lazuli:** enhances communication with the higher self and with spirit guides
- **Malachite:** reveals subconscious blocks, hastens labor and should not be worn until labor begins, brings success, aids in weight reduction
- **Moonstone:** restores harmony in relationships, calms emotions, and induces lucid dreams; is associated with wishes, intuition, and new beginnings

- **Mother of pearl:** brings wealth and protection (especially to new babies)
- **Obsidian:** connects the mind with emotions, grounds spiritual energy into the physical plane, absorbs and disperses negative energies, reduces stress, helps clear subconscious blocks, brings an understanding of the value of silence
- **Onyx:** protects against negative energies and brings emotional stability
- **Opal:** offers inspiration and insight, is a visionary stone
- **Pearl:** purifies, brings clarity and grace
- **Pumice:** eases childbirth, gives protection, helps with banishment
- **Pyrite:** strengthens will, offers a more positive outlook on life, enhances the emotional body, supports one's ability to work with others harmoniously, is associated with practicality
- **Quartz, crystal:** aids with lactation; brings clarity, protection, and healing; enhances psychic ability and personal power
- **Quartz, rose:** helps with all matters of love; brings relaxation and compassion; heals the heart
- **Rhodochrosite:** restores balance in life, helps stabilize emotions, strengthens identity
- **Sapphire:** dispels confusion; promotes fidelity; protects health; attracts money; heals and carries unconditional love; offers peace and balance; relieves emotional pain; magnifies positive intentions; focuses group energy; is associated with blessings, love, and bliss
- **Silver:** provides nourishment and growth; conducts physical and spiritual energy; is associated with the feminine nature of energy, water, the moon, and the subconscious

- **Sodalite:** dispels fear and guilt, stills the mind, relaxes the body, calms inner turmoil
- **Tigereye:** creates courage and confidence, enhances personal power and will, has grounding properties
- **Tourmaline:** brings discernment and vitality; has grounding, healing and protective properties
- **Tourmaline, green:** absorbs negativity, brings success
- **Tourmaline, pink:** induces peaceful sleep
- **Turquoise:** attracts friends; creates joy and an even temper; enhances creative expression; brings peace of mind, emotional balance, friendship, communication, and loyalty; is the color of laughter

GENERAL OBJECT SYMBOLISM

Many objects you see every day represent qualities that can support ritual work:

- **Acorn:** self-potential, great power from humble beginnings
- **Apple:** health, vitality, earth magic, grounding, knowledge
- **Ash:** spiritual purification, essence
- **Ball:** wholeness, unity
- **Balloon:** unrestrained joy, new heights, surrender to the winds of change
- **Beach:** border between the conscious and subconscious (water represents our emotions; earth represents our physicality), balance in life, purification, rejuvenation
- **Beetle:** good luck
- **Bell:** personal attunement, positive energy
- **Bird:** strength coupled with fragility, freedom, messages to and from Spirit, East (air)

- **Bird's nest:** new beginnings, incubation of ideas, spring
- **Boat:** journey, emotional "body"
- **Book:** wisdom, knowledge
- **Bridge:** change, transition, connection
- **Bubble:** joy, exuberance, lightness of being, unburdening
- **Bud:** new life, potential
- **Candle:** light, connection to Spirit, inner fire or spirit, attracting negative or discordant energy
- **Cave:** the unconscious, a place of spiritual retreat, renewal, rebirth, entrance to the subconscious, inner and primordial realms of self
- **Chain:** strength created by union
- **Circle:** unity, strength, protection, infinity, spirituality, wholeness, balance, never-ending cycle of life, death and rebirth, beginnings and endings, Wheel of the Year, Wheel of Life, four directions, four elements
- **Dragon:** life force, great potency, transcendence, personal power, South (fire)
- **Egg:** fertility, new life, birth, mysticism, ancient questions, the sacred, safe container for spiritual transformation (the alchemical egg)
- **Eye:** clarity, truth, vision
- **Fairy:** inner magic
- **Feather:** messages, honesty, East (air)
- **Fire:** purification, initiation, transmutation, South (fire)
- **Fish:** Christianity—Christ was the "fisher of men," spiritual food, renewal, rebirth, West (water)
- **Flower:** beauty, unfolding
- **Key:** opening of doors, solutions close at hand
- **Leaves, green:** growth, abundance, vitality
- **Leaves, turning or brown:** completion, letting go or releasing

133

- **Mandala:** harmony, beauty, balance, self as part of the universe
- **Mermaid:** connection with the sea, emotions, West (water)
- **Mirror:** self-contemplation, reflecting or dispelling unfavorable influences
- **Moon:** feminine (receptive) energy, intuitive nature, tides, fertility, germination of seeds, a woman's moon time (period of menstruation),
- **Nakedness:** freedom, honesty, vulnerability
- **Navel:** connection to mother, personal center, center of the universe
- **Oyster:** hidden treasures, transforming irritations into gifts of great beauty
- **Pinecone:** new life
- **Ring:** completion, wholeness, unity, friendship, eternal love
- **Rock:** strength, endurance, solidity, grounding, North (earth)
- **Salt:** cleansing, purification, dispelling negativity, strength, stability
- **Scissors:** cutting away, releasing, change
- **Seeds:** potential, great things from small beginnings
- **Shell:** protection, West (water)
- **Shoe:** female sex organ, abundance of children
- **Smoke:** visual prayer, cleansing
- **Spiral:** transformation, evolution
- **Star:** guidance, insight
- **Sun:** masculine (projective) energy, power, strength, warmth, light force, clarity, South (fire)
- **Sword:** power, truth, honor, slaying ego, cutting through illusion

- **Thread:** karma or fate, connection to Spirit, Self, friends, community
- **Train:** inner power, attaining goals
- **Tree:** life development, family, connections
- **Wings:** personal freedom, transformation

HERB SYMBOLISM

Herbs, with either medicinal or magical properties, can support us in many ways:

- **Aloe:** beauty, protection, success, peace
- **Anise:** protection, purification, awareness, joy
- **Basil:** protection, love, wealth, healing relationships, courage, fertility, fidelity
- **Bloodroot:** vitality, healing
- **Borage:** courage
- **Cardamom:** strong unions and partnerships
- **Catnip:** joy, friendship, rest
- **Chamomile:** centering, peace, protection, healing
- **Chives:** protection, breaking bad habits
- **Cinnamon:** spiritual quest, power, love, success, safety, healing, protection, happy home
- **Clove:** stolen kisses, fun, love, dispelling negativity, seeing through illusions, protection, money
- **Comfrey:** healing
- **Coriander:** protection of home, peace, longevity, love, security, well-being, intelligence
- **Dandelion:** divination, welcoming, messages, foresight, oracles
- **Dill:** protection of children
- **Elder:** sleep, prosperity, luck, fidelity
- **Eucalyptus:** healing, cleansing, protection

- **Fennel seed:** purification, protection, healing, prosperity
- **Garlic:** protection, healing, courage
- **Ginger:** vibrant energy, zeal, cleansing, health, power, success, love
- **Ginseng:** love, wishes, beauty, desire
- **Hawthorne:** happiness, prosperity, protection, attracting fairies
- **Lavender:** sleep, long life, wishes, peace, protection, love, friendship, spiritual vision, comfort
- **Lemon verbena:** purification, love, blessings
- **Lilac:** clarity, productivity, spiritual balance
- **Marshmallow:** love, protection, dispelling negativity
- **Mint:** money, healing, strength, power
- **Myrrh:** blessing objects, energy, spiritual growth, focus
- **Nettle:** averting danger, protection, healing
- **Parsley:** victory, desires, protection, luck, breaking old habits, protection from accidents
- **Pepper, black:** cleansing, purification, protection, banishing
- **Pepper, white:** mystical transformation
- **Pine:** spiritual clarity, purification, centering, cleansing, healing, productivity
- **Raspberry leaf, red:** strength, nourishment, breast milk production
- **Rose petals:** love, friendship, luck, protection
- **Rosebuds:** new life
- **Rosemary:** bonding, healing, sleep, purification, cleansing, protection, clear thinking, youth, improving memory
- **Sage:** longevity, wishes, wisdom, fertility
- **Saint-John's-wort:** love, joy, protection against ghosts
- **Thyme:** sleep, psychic energy, courage, healing

- **Valerian:** love, calmness, sleep
- **Willow:** protection, love
- **Witch hazel:** protection, chastity, healing, the heart
- **Yarrow:** courage, love, psychic abilities

NUMBER SYMBOLISM

Each number, from one through thirteen, has a unique symbolic value:

- **One:** independence, birth; establishes a starting point
- **Two:** balance, partnership; establishes a connection between two points
- **Three:** sacred diversity (maiden, mother, crone; father, son, holy spirit; the three graces; and so on); establishes a pattern, first group of three in numerology
- **Four:** security, foundation, manifestation
- **Five:** freedom, change, the chaos of creativity
- **Six:** self-harmony, generosity, reliability, second group of three in numerology
- **Seven:** inner wisdom, birth and rebirth, magic
- **Eight:** infinity, energy, personal change, authority, organization
- **Nine:** service to others, endings, completion, last group of three in numerology
- **Ten:** inner voice of reason, transition, the unformed
- **Eleven:** intuition, clairvoyance, spiritual healing, mastery
- **Twelve:** fruitfulness, durability, one full year
- **Thirteen:** devotion, patience, convictions

135

TREE SYMBOLISM

Trees possess qualities that can support your ritual:

- **Apple:** knowledge, success, healing
- **Aspen:** dispelling fear
- **Birch:** Mother Earth, balance, releasing old ideas
- **Cedar:** inner potential, cleansing, healing
- **Elm:** overcoming weaknesses by turning them into strengths
- **Fig:** enlightenment, awakening intuition and creative forces within, releasing blockages
- **Hazel:** peace, wisdom, divination
- **Maple:** balance, grounding
- **Mistletoe:** fertility, protection, luck, dreams
- **Oak:** strength
- **Pine:** purification, cleansing, spiritual clarity, centering, healing, productivity
- **Palm:** freedom, abundance, warmth
- **Redwood:** eldership, time, immortality, perspective, imagination
- **Rowan:** goddess energy, strength, protection, magic
- **Spruce:** balance
- **Walnut:** free spirit, life cycles

Recommended Resources

ANIMAL SYMBOLISM

(See also "Symbolic Gifts" under "Ritual Supplies," below.)

Animal-Speak by Ted Andrews

Medicine Cards: The Discovery of Power through the Ways of Animals by Jamie Sams and David Carson

FEMININE EXPRESSIONS OF THE DIVINE

(See also "Symbolic Gifts" under "Ritual Supplies," below.)

Archangels and Ascended Masters: A Guide to Working and Healing with Divinities and Deities by Doreen Virtue

Celtic Myth and Magick: Harnessing the Power of the Gods and Goddesses by Edain McCoy

Circle Round: Raising Children in Goddess Traditions by Starhawk, Diane Baker, and Anne Hill, www.circle-round.com

Goddesses: An Illustrated Journey into the Myths, Symbols, and Rituals of the Goddess by Manuela Dunn Mascetti

The Grandmother of Time: A Women's Book of Celebrations, Spells and Sacred Objects for Every Month of the Year by Zsuzsanna E. Budapest

Motherpeace: A Way to the Goddess through Myth, Art and Tarot by Vicki Noble, www.motherpeace.com

The New Book of Goddesses and Heroines by Patricia Monaghan

FOOD SYMBOLISM AND RECIPES

Goddess in the Kitchen by Marjorie Lapanja

A Kitchen Witch's Cookbook by Patricia Telesco6

The Wicca Cookbook: Recipes, Ritual, Lore by Jamie Wood and Tara Seefeldt

Witch in the Kitchen: Magical Cooking for All Seasons by Cait Johnson

HERBS

(See also "Herb Farms and Bulk Herbs" under "Ritual Supplies," below.)

All books by Rosemary Gladstar, www.sagemountain.com

The Star Herbal by Robert Menzies

Wise Woman Herbal for the Childbearing Year by Susun Weed, www.susunweed.com

MEDITATION AND VISUALIZATION

Birthing from Within: An Extra-Ordinary Guide to Child birth Preparation by Pam England and Rob Horowitz, www.birthingfromwithin.com

Celebrating Motherhood: A Comforting Companion for Every Mother (originally published as *Mother's Nature*) by Andrea Alban Gosline and Lisa Burnett Bossi

Creative Visualization by Shakti Gawain

The Dance by Oriah Mountain Dreamer, www.oriahmountaindreamer.com

The Invitation by Oriah Mountain Dreamer, www.oriahmountaindreamer.com

Mother Wit by Diane Mariechild. Note: Hard to find; check Amazon.com's used booksellers, www.amazon.com

The Pregnant Woman's Comfort Book: A Self-Nurturing Guide to Your Emotional Well-Being during Pregnancy and Early Motherhood by Jennifer Louden, www.comfortqueen.com

The Woman's Comfort Book: A Self-Nurturing Guide for Restoring Balance to Your Life by Jennifer Louden, www.comfortqueen.com

MEHNDI

(See also "Mehndi Supplies" under "Ritual Supplies.")

WEBSITE

The Reverend Bunny's Secret Henna Diary http://reverndbunny.sphosting.com.

BOOKS

The Art of Mehndi by Sumita Batra

Mehndi: The Art of Henna Body Painting by Carine Fabius

Traditional Mehndi Designs: A Treasury of Henna Body Art by Dorine Van Den Beukel

MOVEMENT

Sweat Your Prayers: Movement as Spiritual Practice by Gabrielle Roth, www.gabrielleroth.com

MUSICAL RESOURCES

BOOKS AND SONGBOOKS

Circle Round: Raising Children in Goddess Traditions by Starhawk, Diane Baker, and Anne Hill, www.circle-round.com. See also *Circle Round and Sing* CD by Anne Hill.

The Heart of the Circle: A Guide to Drumming by Holly Blue Hawkins

Rise Up Singing: The Group Singing Songbook edited by Peter Blood and Annie Patterson, 1-888-746-4688

Songs for Earthlings: A Green Spirituality Songbook compiled by Julie Forest Middleton

RECORDED MUSIC

To hear music samples, try www.amazon.com or the individual artist's website.

Adiemus by Adiemus. Female vocals, tribal rhythms: ethereal, meditative, upbeat.

Bones (or) Trance by Gabrielle Roth and the Mirrors. Instrumentals: from meditative to tribal dance.

Canyon Trilogy by R. Carlos Nakai. Native American flute: meditative, reflective.

The Celtic Cradle by Jill Rogoff. Celtic female vocals: lullabies, lyrical.

A Circle Is Cast by Libana. Women's songs and chants.

Circle of Women produced by Alice Di Micele. Women's songs and chants.

Circle Round and Sing by Anne Hill, www.circleround.com. Female vocals: earth-based songs and chants. See also *Circle Round* book for words and music.

Embrace (or) The Essence by Deva Premal. Female vocals, ancient mantras, reflective rhythms: from meditative to upbeat/dance.

Exotica—World Music Divas compilation of various artists. Female vocals, music from many cultures and traditions: from reflective to upbeat.

From the Goddess/O Great Spirit by Robert Gass and On the Wings of Song. Earth-based songs and chants.

In Search of Angels compilation of various artists. Instrumental and vocal: meditative, ethereal, lyrical.

In the Arms of the Wild by Beverly Frederick. Women's earth-based songs and chants.

Ladyslipper Music by Women. Music catalog, www.ladyslipper.org, 1-800-634-6044.

The Mask and the Mirror by Loreena McKennitt. Celtic female vocals: from meditative to upbeat and dance.

Music to Be Born By by Mickey Hart. Infant heartbeat and percussion: reflective, upbeat.

Offerings (or) Sunyata by Vas. Female vocals, ethnic fusion: from reflective to upbeat.

Pacific Moon I, II, III compilation of various artists. New music based on Asian cultures and traditions.

Putamayo Presents . . . compilations of various artists. Folk music collections from many cultures and traditions: instrumentals and vocals in a wide range of styles.

Quiet Mind by Nawang Khechog. Tibetan bamboo flute: meditative, lyrical.

Returning (or) Praises for the World by Jennifer Berezen. Female vocals: transformational, a journey in itself.

Silent Joy by Anugama (Werner Hagen). Pan flute: reflective, meditative, lyrical.

Siren Song by Connemara. Celtic female vocals: reflective.

Voices on the Eastern Wind (or) the Vine (or) Nectar by Kitka. Female vocals: Eastern European folk songs, beautiful and powerful!

Watermark (or) Shepherd Moons by Enya. Celtic female vocals: reflective.

Weaving My Ancestors' Voices by Sheila Chandra. Anglo-Indian female vocals, blend of modern and traditional music: from reflective to upbeat.

Yoga Trance Dance by Shiva Rea, Geoffrey Gordon, and Ben Leinbach. Guided meditation and guided dance music, plus additional all-instrumental disc.

PARENTING

MAGAZINE

Mothering Magazine, www.mothering.com, 1-800-984-8116

BOOKS

The Baby Book by William Sears, M.D., and Martha
Sears, R.N., www.askdrsears.com

Chinaberry. Book and gift catalog, www.chinaberry.com,
1-800-776-2242

Everyday Blessings by Myla and Jon Kabat-Zinn

Mitten Strings for God: Reflections for Mothers in a Hurry
by Katrina Kenison

Raising Your Spirited Child by Mary Sheedy Kurcinka

The Seven Spiritual Laws of Parenting by Deepak Chopra

Spiritual Parenting by Gayle and Hugh Prather

POEMS, PRAYERS, AND READINGS

*Celebrating Motherhood: A Comforting Companion for Every
Mother* (Originally published as *Mother's Nature*) by
Andrea Alban Gosline and Lisa Burnett Bossi

Circle of Stones: Woman's Journey to Herself by Judith Duerk

Circle Round: Raising Children in Goddess Traditions by
Starhawk, Diane Baker, and Anne Hill,
www.circleround.com

I Hear Your Name: Poems That Nurture and Empower by
Lela Florel, www.lelaearthspirit.com

Illuminata by Marianne Williamson, www.marianne.com

*I Sit Listening to the Wind: Woman's Encounter within
Herself* by Judith Duerk

*Seven Times the Sun: Guiding Your Child through the
Rhythms of the Day* by Shea Darian

POSTPARTUM SUPPORT

ORGANIZATIONS

La Leche League International (LLLI),
www.lalecheleague.org, 1-800-LALECHE
(525-3243). Breastfeeding support.

National Association of Postpartum Care Services
(NAPCS), www.napcs.org, 1-800-453-6852.
Postpartum doula association.

BOOKS

*After the Baby's Birth… A Woman's Way to Wellness: A
Complete Guide for Postpartum Women* by Robin Lim

The Womanly Art of Breastfeeding 6th ed., by La Leche
League International, www.lalecheleague.org

PREGNANCY AND CHILDBIRTH

ORGANIZATIONS

Birthing the Future, www.birthingthefuture.com,
970-884-4090. Childbirth education.

Birth Works, www.birthworks.org, 1-888-TO BIRTH
(862-4784). Childbirth education and doula services.

DONA International, www.dona.org, 1-888-788-DONA
(3662). Birth support doulas.

Global Maternal/Child Health Association (GMCHA)
and Waterbirth International, www.waterbirth.org,
1-800-641-2229. Pregnancy, childbirth and parenting
support, rental, and use of portable tubs for water births.

Midwives Alliance of North America (MANA),
www.mana.org, 1-888-923-MANA (6262). Midwives
association.

MAGAZINE

Mothering Magazine, www.mothering.com,
1-800-984-8116

BOOKS

Birthing from Within: An Extra-Ordinary Guide to Child birth Preparation by Pam England and Rob Horowitz, www.birthingfromwithin.com

The Birth Partner: Everything You Need to Know to Help a Woman through Childbirth by Penny Simpkin

Celebrating Motherhood: A Comforting Companion for Every Mother (Originally published as *Mother's Nature*) by Andrea Alban Gosline and Lisa Burnett Bossi

Conscious Conception (or) Hygieia (or) Prenatal Yoga by Jeannine Parvati Baker

Gentle Birth Choices by Barbara Harper, www.water birth.org. Book and video on natural and water births.

Immaculate Deception II: Myth, Magic, and Birth by Suzanne Arms, www.birthingthefuture.com

The Natural Pregnancy Book by Aviva Jill Romm

The Pregnancy Book: A Month-by-Month Guide by William Sears, M.D., and Martha Sears, R.N., www.askdrsears.com

The Pregnant Woman's Comfort Book: A Self-Nurturing Guide to Your Emotional Well-Being during Pregnancy and Early Motherhood by Jennifer Louden, www.comfortqueen.com

Spiritual Midwifery by Ina May Gaskin, www.inamay.com

RITUAL

The 13 Original Clan Mothers by Jamie Sams

Blessingways: A Guide to Mother-Centered Baby Showers by Shari Maser, www.blessingway.net

Casting the Circle: A Women's Book of Ritual by Diane Stein

Celtic Myth and Magick: Harnessing the Power of the Gods and Goddesses by Edain McCoy

The Circle Is Sacred: A Medicine Book for Women by Scout Cloud Lee

Circle Round: Raising Children in Goddess Traditions by Starhawk, Diane Baker, and Anne Hill, www.circle-round.com

Creating Circles of Power and Magic: Harnessing the Power of the Gods and Goddesses by Caitlin Libera

Fire in the Head: Shamanism and the Celtic Spirit by Tom Cowan

The Grandmother of Time: A Women's Book of Celebrations, Spells and Sacred Objects for Every Month of the Year by Zsuzsanna E. Budapest

Jambalaya: The Natural Woman's Book of Personal Charms and Practical Rituals by Luisah Teish

The Joy of Ritual: Spiritual Recipes to Celebrate Milestones, Ease Transitions, and Make Every Day Sacred by Barbara Biziou

Practicing the Presence of the Goddess: Everyday Rituals to Transform Your World by Barbara Ardinger

To Ride a Silver Broomstick: New Generation Witchcraft by Silver RavenWolf

A Woman's Book of Rituals and Celebrations by Barbara Ardinger

The Woman's Comfort Book: A Self-Nurturing Guide for Restoring Balance to Your Life by Jennifer Louden, www.comfortqueen.com

The Woman's Retreat Book: A Guide to Restoring, Rediscovering, and Reawakening Your True Self—in a Moment, an Hour, a Day, or a Weekend by Jennifer Louden, www.comfortqueen.com

Women's Rituals: A Sourcebook by Barbara Walker

RITUAL SUPPLIES

BELLY CASTING SUPPLIES
Proud Body, www.proudbody.com, 1-877-972-1859

CANDLES
Gifts of Nature, www.giftsofnaturereps.com,
   1-800-733-7783
Beyond the Rainbow, www.rainbowcrystal.com,
   1-888-480-3529
Scents and Sprays, www.scentsandsprays.com,
   1-702-515-2058

HERB FARMS AND BULK HERBS
Jean's Greens, www.jeansgreens.com, 1-888-845-8327
Healing Spirits Herb Farm and Education Center,
   www.infoblvd.net/healingspirits/, 1-607-566-2701
Lavender Moon Herb Gardens, www.lavendermoon
   herbs.com, 1-585-624-4220
Mountain Rose Herbs, www.mountainroseherbs.com,
   1-800-879-3337

JEWELRY-MAKING SUPPLIES
Bead Studio, www.beadstudio.com, 1-541-488-3037
Beadworks. www.beadworks.com, 1-800-232-3761
Fire Mountain Gems and Beads,
   www.firemountaingems.com, 1-800-423-2319

MEHNDI SUPPLIES
(See also "Mehndi," above.)
Earth Henna, www.earthhenna.com, 1-323-460-7333
Mehndi Skin Art Distributor, www.mehndiskinart.com,
   1-250-370-9337

SMUDGE STICKS
Eye of the Day, www.eyeoftheday.com, 1-800-631-4603
Matoska Trading Company, www.matoska.com,
   1-800-926-6286

MASSAGE AND ROSE ESSENTIAL OILS
Escential Lotions and Oils, www.escentialonline.com,
   1-866-947-6666
Nanda Essential Oils, www.nandaoils.com,
   1-916-455-1512

STATUARY
Mythic Images, www.mythicimages.com,
   1-707-795-8047
Sacred Source, www.sacredsource.com, 1-800-290-6203

SYMBOLIC GIFTS
Beyond the Rainbow, www.rainbowcrystal.com,
   1-888-480-3529. Animal talisman stones.
Lela Earth Spirit Arts, www.lelaearthspirit.com. Hand
   made jewelry, poetry book, prints, and wall hangings.
yOni, www.yoni.com. You should just see for yourself.

YARN
Halcyon Yarn, www.halcyonyarn.com, 1-800-341-0282
The Yarn Market, www.yarnmarket.com, 1-888-996-9276
Yarnia, The Yarn Universe, www.yarnia.com,
   1-800-435-4522

SACRED SPACE
Altars Made Easy by Peg Streep

Home Sanctuary: Practical Ways to Create a Spiritually Fulfilling Environment by Nicole Marcelis

Sacred Space by Denise Linn, www.deniselinn.com

Space Clearing: How to Purify and Create Harmony in Your Home by Denise Linn, www.deniselinn.com

SYMBOLISM

The Secret Language of Signs by Denise Linn, www.deniselinn.com

The Urban Pagan: Magical Living in a 9-to-5 World by Patricia Telesco

The Woman's Encyclopedia of Symbols and Sacred Objects by Barbara G. Walker

WOMEN'S SPIRITUALITY

ORGANIZATIONS

Woman Within International, www.womanwithin.org. Helps women discover the power of who they are through intensive weekend training.

BOOKS

Aphrodite's Daughters: Women's Sexual Stories and the Journey of the Soul by Jalaja Bonheim, www.jalajabonheim.com

Casting the Circle: A Women's Book of Ritual by Diane Stein

The Circle Is Sacred: A Medicine Book for Women by Scout Cloud Lee

The Circle of Life: Thirteen Archetypes for Every Woman by Elizabeth Davis and Carol Leonard

Circle of Stones: Woman's Journey to Herself by Judith Duerk

Creating Circles of Power and Magic: Harnessing the Power of the Gods and Goddesses by Caitlin Libera

Everyday Grace: Having Hope, Finding Forgiveness, and Making Miracles by Marianne Williamson, www.marianne.com

The Grandmother of Time: A Women's Book of Celebrations, Spells and Sacred Objects for Every Month of the Year by Zsuzsanna E. Budapest

I Sit Listening to the Wind: Woman's Encounter within Herself by Judith Duerk

The Millionth Circle: How to Change Ourselves and the World: The Essential Guide to Women's Circles by Jean Shinoda Bolen, www.jeanbolen.com

The Rings of Empowerment: A Guide to Discovering and Fulfilling Your Life Purpose as Part of a Co-Creative Team by Carolyn Anderson

Sacred Circles: A Guide to Creating Your Own Women's Spirituality Group by Robin Deen Carnes and Sally Craig

Simple Abundance: A Daybook of Comfort and Joy by Sarah Ban Breathnach, www.simpleabundance.com

Succulent Wild Woman: Dancing with Your Wonder-Full Self by Sark, www.planetsark.com

The Woman's Comfort Book: A Self-Nurturing Guide for Restoring Balance to Your Life by Jennifer Louden, www.comfortqueen.com

The Woman's Retreat Book: A Guide to Restoring, Rediscovering, and Reawakening Your True Self—in a Moment, an Hour, a Day, or a Weekend by Jennifer Louden, www.comfortqueen.com

A Woman's Worth by Marianne Williamson, www.marianne.com

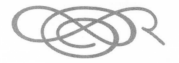

Books

Anderson, Carolyn. *The Rings of Empowerment: A Guide to Discovering and Fulfilling Your Life Purpose as Part of a Co-Creative Team.* San Anselmo, CA: Global Family, 1993.

Andrews, Ted. *Animal-Speak: The Spiritual and Magical Powers of Creatures Great and Small.* St. Paul: Llewllyn Publications, 2000.

Ardinger, Barbara. *A Women's Book of Rituals and Celebrations.* rev. ed. Novato, CA: New World Library, 1995.

Argüelles, José, and Miriam Argüelles. *Mandala.* Boulder: Shambhala Publications, 1972.

Arrien, Angeles. *The Four-Fold Way: Walking the Paths of the Warrior, Teacher, Healer, and Visionary.* New York: HarperSanFrancisco, 1993.

Babcock, Michael. *Susan Seddon Boulet: The Goddess Paintings.* San Francisco: Pomegranate Artbooks, 1994.

Ban Breathnach, Sarah. *Simple Abundance: A Daybook of Comfort and Joy.* New York: Warner Books, Inc., 1995.

———. *Something More: Excavating Your Authentic Self.* New York: Warner Books, Inc., 1998.

Batra, Sumita, with Liz Wilde. *The Art of Mehndi.* New York: Penguin Studio, 1999.

Beck, Renee, and Sydney Barbara Metrick. *The Art of Ritual: A Guide to Creating and Performing Your Own Rituals for Growth and Change.* Berkeley: Celestial Arts, 1990.

Bolen, Jean Shinoda. *Goddesses in Everywoman: A New Psychology of Women.* New York: Harper & Row Publishers, Inc., 1984.

———. *The Millionth Circle: How to Change Ourselves and the World: The Essential Guide to Women's Circles.* Berkeley: Conari Press, 1999.

Bonheim, Jalaja. *Aphrodite's Daughters: Women's Sexual Stories and the Journey of the Soul.* New York: Fireside, 1997.

Budapest, Zsuzsanna E. *The Grandmother of Time: A Women's Book of Celebrations, Spells, and Sacred Objects for Every Month of the Year.* New York: HarperSanFrancisco, 1989.

Campanelli, Pauline. *Pagan Rites of Passage.* St. Paul: Llewellyn Publications, 1998.

Carnes, Robin Deen, and Sally Craig. *Sacred Circles: A Guide to Creating Your Own Women's Spirituality Group.* New York: HarperSanFrancisco, 1998.

Darian, Shea. *Seven Times the Sun: Guiding Your Child through the Rhythms of the Day.* Marshall, WI: Gilead Press, 2001.

Dreamer, Oriah Mountain. *The Dance.* New York: HarperSanFrancisco, 2001.

———. *The Invitation.* New York: HarperSanFrancisco, 1999.

Dunham, Carroll, and others. *Mamatoto: A Celebration of Birth.* New York: Penguin Books, 1993.

Duerk, Judith. *Circle of Stones: Woman's Journey to Herself.* Philadelphia: Innisfree Press, Inc., 1989.

Eagle, Brooke Medicine. *Buffalo Woman Comes Singing.* New York: Ballantine Books, 1991.

England, Pam, and Rob Horowitz. *Birthing from Within: An Extra-Ordinary Guide to Childbirth Preparation.* Albuquerque: Partera Press, 1998.

Erdrich, Louise. *The Blue Jay's Dance.* New York: HarperCollins Publishers, 1995.

Fabius, Carine. *Mehndi: The Art of Henna Body Painting.* New York: Three Rivers Press, 1998.

Fields, Rick, Peggy Taylor, Rex Weyler, and Rick Ingrasci. *Chop Wood, Carry Water: A Guide to Finding Spiritual Fulfillment in Everyday Life.* Edited by *New Age Journal.* Los Angeles: Jeremy P. Tarcher, Inc., 1984.

Fix, William R. *Star Maps: Astounding New Evidence from Ancient Civilisations and Modern Scientific Research of Man's Origins and Return to the Stars.* Toronto: Jonathan-James Books, 1979.

Florel, Lela. *I Hear Your Name: Poems That Nurture and Empower.* Fairfield, CT: Earth Spirit Press, 1995.

Gosline, Andrea Alban, and Lisa Burnett Bossi. *Celebrating Motherhood: A Comforting Companion for Every Expecting Mother.* Berkeley: Conari Press, 2002. Originally published as *Mother's Nature: Timeless Wisdom for the Journey into Motherhood.* Berkeley: Conari Press, 1999.

Grinnan, Jeanne Brinkman, and others. *Sisters of the Thirteen Moons: Rituals Celebrating Women's Lives.* Webster, NY: Prism Collective, 1996.

Hall, Manly P. *The Secret Teachings of All Ages: An Encyclopedic Outline of Masonic, Hermetic, Qabbalistic and Rosicrucian Symbolical Philosophy.* Los Angeles: The Philosophical Research Society, Inc., 1988.

Hawkins, Holly Blue. *The Heart of the Circle: A Guide to Drumming.* Freedom, CA: The Crossing Press, 1999.

Huston, River. *The Goddess Within.* Philadelphia: Running Press, 1999.

Huxley, Francis. *The Way of the Sacred: The Rites and Symbols, Beliefs and Tabus, That Men Have Held in Awe and Wonder, through the Ages.* Garden City, NY: Doubleday and Company, Inc., 1974.

Johnsen, Linda. *Daughters of the Goddess: The Women Saints of India.* St. Paul: Yes International Publishers, 1994.

Kabat-Zinn, Myla, and Jon Kabat-Zinn. *Everyday Blessings: The Inner Work of Mindful Parenting.* New York: Hyperion, 1997.

Lake-Thom, Bobby. *Spirits of the Earth: A Guide to Native American Nature Symbols, Stories, and Ceremonies.* New York: Plume, 1997.

La Leche League International. *The Womanly Art of Breastfeeding.* 6th ed. Edited by Judy Torgus and Gwen Gotsch. Schaumburg, IL: La Leche League International, 1997.

Lapanja, Margie. *Goddess in the Kitchen: 210 Heavenly Recipes, Spirited Stories and Saucy Secrets.* Berkeley: Conari Press, 1998.

Lee, Scout Cloud. *The Circle Is Sacred: A Medicine Book for Women.* Tulsa: Council Oak Books, 1994.

Libera, Caitlin. *Creating Circles of Power and Magic: A Women's Guide to Sacred Community.* Freedom, CA: The Crossing Press, 1994.

Lim, Robin. *After the Baby's Birth, A Woman's Way to Wellness: A Complete Guide for Postpartum Women.* Berkeley: Celestial Arts, 1991.

Lindbergh, Anne Morrow. *Gift from the Sea.* New York: Pantheon Books, 1983.

Linn, Denise. *Sacred Space: Clearing and Enhancing the Energy of Your Home.* New York: Ballantine Books, 1995.

———. *The Secret Language of Signs.* New York: Ballantine Books, 1996.

———. *Space Clearing: How to Purify and Create Harmony in Your Home.* Chicago: Contemporary Books, 2000.

Louden, Jennifer. *The Pregnant Woman's Comfort Book: A Self-Nurturing Guide to Your Emotional Well-Being during Pregnancy and Early Motherhood.* New York: Harper SanFrancisco, 1995.

———. *The Woman's Comfort Book: A Self-Nurturing Guide for Restoring Balance in Your Life.* New York: HarperSanFrancisco, 1992.

———. *The Woman's Retreat Book: A Guide to Restoring, Rediscovering, and Reawakening Your True Self—in a Moment, an Hour, a Day, or a Weekend.* New York: HarperSanFrancisco, 1997.

Marcelis, Nicole. *Home Sanctuary: Practical Ways to Create a Spiritually Fulfilling Environment.* Chicago: Contemporary Books, 2001.

Mariechild, Diane. *Mother Wit: A Feminist Guide to Psychic Development.* Trumansburg, NY: The Crossing Press, 1981.

Marks, Kate. *Circle of Song: Songs, Chants, and Dances for Ritual and Celebration.* rev. ed. Amherst, MA: Full Circle Press, 1999.

Martin, Stella. *Space Clearing: The Ancient Art of Purifying, Cleansing, and Harmonizing Your Living Space.* London: Lorenz Books, 2002.

Mascetti, Manuela Dunn. *Goddesses: An Illustrated Journey into the Myths, Symbols, and Rituals of the Goddess.* New York: Barnes & Noble Books, 1998.

McCoy, Edain. *Celtic Myth and Magick: Harnessing the Power of the Gods and Goddesses.* St. Paul: Llewellyn Publications, 1999.

Middleton, Julie Forest. *Songs for Earthlings: A Green Spirituality Songbook.* Philadelphia: Emerald Earth Publishing, 1998.

Mitchell, Rosemary Catalano. *Birthings and Blessings: Liberating Worship Services for the Inclusive Church.* New York: Crossroad, 1991.

Monaghan, Patricia. *The New Book of Goddesses and Heroines.* St. Paul: Llewellyn Publications, 2000.

Moore, Thomas, ed. *The Education of the Heart: Readings and Sources for Care of the Soul, Soul Mates, and the Re-Enchantment of Everyday Life.* New York: Harper-Collins, 1996.

Noble, Vicki. *Motherpeace: A Way to the Goddess through Myth, Art and Tarot.* New York: HarperCollins, 1994.

Northup, Lesley A. *Ritualizing Women: Patterns of Spirituality.* Cleveland: Pilgrim Press, 1997.

Pollack, Rachel. *The Power of Ritual.* The Omega Institute Mind, Body, Spirit Series. New York: Dell Publishing, 2000.

Randour, Mary Lou. *Women's Psyche, Women's Spirit: The Reality of Relationships.* New York: Columbia University Press, 1987.

RavenWolf, Silver. *Silver's Spells for Protection.* St. Paul: Llewellyn Publications, 2000.

Romm, Aviva Jill. *The Natural Pregnancy Book.* Freedom,

CA: The Crossing Press, 1997.

Roth, Gabrielle. *Sweat Your Prayers: Movement as Spiritual Practice*. New York: Putnam Books, 1997.

Sams, Jamie. *Dancing the Dream: The Seven Sacred Paths of Human Transformation*. New York: HarperSanFrancisco, 1998.

Sams, Jamie, and David Carson. *Medicine Cards: The Discovery of Power through the Ways of Animals*. Santa Fe: Bear & Company, 1988.

Sark. *Succulent Wild Woman: Dancing with Your Wonder-Full Self.* New York: Fireside Books, 1997.

Sered, Susan Starr. *Priestess, Mother, Sacred Sister: Religions Dominated by Women*. Oxford: Oxford University Press, 1994.

Simkin, Penny. *The Birth Partner: Everything You Need to Know to Help a Woman through Childbirth*. Boston: The Harvard Common Press, 1989.

Starhawk, Diane Baker, and Anne Hill. *Circle Round: Raising Children in Goddess Traditions*. New York: Bantam Books, 1998.

Stassinopoulos, Agapi. *Conversations with the Goddesses: Revealing the Divine Power within You*. New York: Stewart, Tabori & Chang, 1999.

Stein, Diane. *Casting the Circle: A Women's Book of Ritual*. Freedom, CA: The Crossing Press, 1990.

Streep, Peg. *Altars Made Easy: A Complete Guide to Creating Your Own Sacred Space*. New York: HarperSanFrancisco, 1997.

Teish, Luisah. *Jambalaya: The Natural Woman's Book of Personal Charms and Practical Rituals*. New York: HarperSanFrancisco, 1985.

Telesco, Patricia. *A Kitchen Witch's Cookbook*. St. Paul: Llewllyn Publications, 1994.

———. *The Urban Pagan: Magical Living in a 9-to-5 World*. St. Paul: Llewllyn Publications, 1997.

Van Den Beukel, Dorine. *Traditional Mehndi Designs: A Treasury of Henna Body Art*. Boston: Shambhala Publications, 2000.

Virtue, Doreen. *Archangels and Ascended Masters: A Guide to Working and Healing with Divinities and Deities*. Carlsbad, CA: Hay House, Inc., 2003.

Vogel, Karen, and Vicki Noble. *Motherpeace Tarot Guidebook*. Stamford, CT: U.S. Game Systems, Inc., 1995.

Walker, Barbara G. *The Woman's Encyclopedia of Myths and Secrets*. New York: HarperSanFrancisco, 1983.

———. *Women's Rituals: A Sourcebook*. New York: Harper & Row Publishers, 1990.

Weed, Susun S. *Wise Woman Herbal for the Childbearing Year*. Woodstock, NY: Ash Tree Publishing, 1986.

Williamson, Marianne. *Everyday Grace: Having Hope, Finding Forgiveness, and Making Miracles*. New York: Riverhead Books, 2002.

———. *Illuminata: A Return to Prayer*. New York: Riverhead Books, 1995.

Wood, Jamie, and Tara Seefeldt. *The Wicca Cookbook: Recipes, Rituals, Lore*. Berkeley: Celestial Arts, 2000.

Wyman, Leland C. *Blessingway*. Tucson: The University of Arizona Press, 1970.

Articles and Pamphlets

Burke, Cynthia. *A Blessingway.* Wakefield, RI: Greenwood Press, 1994.

Herring, Lucinda. *Celebration of the Mother: Blessingways for Women Giving Birth.* Spring Valley, CA: Chinaberry Books, Inc., 1997.

Lang, Raven. *Blessingway into Birth: A Rite of Passage.* Santa Cruz, CA: Raven Lang, 1995.

Sweet, Gail Grenier. "Blessingway." *Mothering Magazine,* (Winter 1982): 99–101.

INDEX

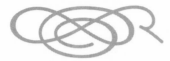

H

Hair
    braiding and beading, 64
    brushing, 63
Ham-and-Spinach Bread Pudding, 90
Hathor, 124
Headpieces, 62, 68
Hera, 124
Herbs
    footbath of, 63
    resources for, 137
    sources of, 141
    symbolism of, 134–35
Hestia, 124
Honoring, 59–62

I

Invitations, 18–20
Invocation, 37
Irish Soda Bread, 92
Ishtar, 125
Isis, 125
Ix Chel, 125

J

Jewelry
    giving, 68
    making, 70–71, 121, 141
Juno, 125

K

Kuan Yin (Kwan Yin), 45, 125

L

Labor candles, 22
La Leche League, 115, 139
Laying-on-of-hands
    blessing, 73
    ritual, 111–12, 113
Lemonade, Mint, 96
Lemon Pasta Salad with Feta Cheese, 93
Letters to the baby, 62

Lilith, 125
Liminal limbo, 109–11
Location, choosing, 18
Lucina, 125

M

Mami, 125–26
Mary, Virgin, 126
Massage
    oils, 141
    pampering with, 63
Meditation
    guiding, 100
    laying-on-of-hands, 111–12, 113
    music, 52
    resources for, 137
    shell, 52–55
    silent, 51–52
Mehndi, 64, 137, 141
Mint Lemonade, 96
Mobiles, 69
Molasses Postpartum Cookies, 94
Moore, Thomas, 9
Mother Earth, 126
    altar for, 44
    summoning, 46
Mother's Blessing Tea, 96
Mother-to-be
    advice for, 11–12
    ancestors of, 122
    effects of blessingway ritual on, 109
    emotional, 34
    gifts for, 64–68
    in liminal limbo, 109–11
    planning and, 11, 15–16, 17
    questions for, 17
Movement, 29, 137
Muffins, Carrot-Raisin, 87
Music
    books and songbooks, 137
    meditation, 52
    recorded, 29, 137–38

Symbolism
    animal, 127–28, 136
    color, 128
    flower and plant, 128–29
    food, 129–31, 136
    gem and stone, 131–33
    general object, 133–34
    herb, 134–35
    number, 135–36
    resources for, 142
    shell, 131–33
    tree, 136

T

Tamale Pie, 89
Tea, Mother's Blessing, 96
Ten, symbolic value of, 135
Thanks, giving, 81–82
Themes, 26
Thirteen, symbolic value of, 136
Three, symbolic value of, 135
Tone, setting, 51, 103
Traditions, 4, 8. *See also* Rituals
Tree symbolism, 136
Twelve, symbolic value of, 136
Two, symbolic value of, 135

V

Vegetable Stew, African, 91
Venus of Willendorf, 126
Vesta, 126
Virgin Mary, 126
Visualization
    birth story, 52
    guiding, 100
    resources for, 137

W

Web, weaving, 79, 81, 122
West
    altar for, 40
    correspondences for, 38
    qualities of, 39

White, 128
Witches, 9
Women
    circles and, 10
    culture and, 4–5
    ritual and, 7–9
    spirituality and, 9, 142
    as witches, 9
Worry Jar ritual, 56, 122
Wreaths, 62, 68, 121

Y

Yarn
    sources of, 141
    weaving web of, 79, 81
Yellow, 128
Yemaya, 126–27